# THE
# BIG
## PRESCRIPTION

T0117724

# THE
# BIG
# PRESCRIPTION

## Balancing The Three Principles
## Of Enduring Health

# DR. SHAN HUSSAIN

Advantage.

Published by Advantage, Charleston, South Carolina.
Member of Advantage Media Group.

ADVANTAGE is a registered trademark and the Advantage colophon is a trademark of Advantage Media Group, Inc.

Printed in the United States of America.

ISBN: 978-1-59932-716-7
LCCN: 2016962225

Cover design by Damonza and Katie Biondo.

This publication is designed to provide accurate and authoritative information in regard to the subject matter covered. It is sold with the understanding that the publisher is not engaged in rendering legal, accounting, or other professional services. If legal advice or other expert assistance is required, the services of a competent professional person should be sought.

Advantage Media Group is proud to be a part of the Tree Neutral® program. Tree Neutral offsets the number of trees consumed in the production and printing of this book by taking proactive steps such as planting trees in direct proportion to the number of trees used to print books. To learn more about Tree Neutral, please visit **www.treeneutral.com**.

Advantage Media Group is a publisher of business, self-improvement, and professional development books. We help entrepreneurs, business leaders, and professionals share their Stories, Passion, and Knowledge to help others Learn & Grow. Do you have a manuscript or book idea that you would like us to consider for publishing? Please visit **advantagefamily.com** or call **1.866.775.1696.**

*For Emma and Daniel.*

# DISCLAIMER

The content in this book is not intended as a substitute for the medical advice of a primary physician. Please regularly consult with your physician in matters relating to your health, particularly with respect to any symptoms that may require diagnosis or immediate medical attention. Due to the variance of individuals' lifestyles and bodies, the methods elaborated on in this book are not guaranteed to produce your desired result; therefore, the author and publisher do not assume any liability to any party for any loss, damage, or disruption caused by the choice to implement any of the following health strategies.

# TABLE OF CONTENTS

# FOREWORD

I had the honour of meeting Shan a few years ago in Tenerife while teaching Life Mastery, a program designed by Tony Robbins. Fifteen years ago Tony and Sage asked me to launch this program, and I have taught over two hundred of these events and have met thousands of amazing people from around the world. We complete a one-week cleanse that helps people build a strong foundation physically, spiritually, and emotionally. Each week I always acknowledge the healthcare professionals in the room, especially doctors, for coming to see that maybe there are other things that contribute to one's overall health. Many doctors are not even required to take classes in nutrition.

When I met Shan I could tell that he already "got it"—he understood the importance of physical, emotional, and spiritual health and so much more.

*The Big Prescription* is just what is needed to help heal people and is also a great guide for being conscious and mindful. This book gives such practical tools of wisdom and common sense for all. Shan really helps everyone understand the importance of lifestyle choices and how they affect all areas of our lives.

Shan presents an in-depth look to help people understand the importance of creating balance. This book literally is life transforming. It will help you to not only add more years to your life but also more life to your years.

I encourage you to apply what you can. Do what feels right, and remember to always stay true to who you are.

To your health,

**LOREN SLOCUM**
Mom
International Speaker
Author of *No Greater Love, Life Tuneups, Chicken Soup for the Soul: Time to Thrive,* and *The Courage to Raise a Gentleman*

# ACKNOWLEDGMENTS

This book could not have been written without the incredible advice, support, and endless encouragement from so many people that I wish to acknowledge.

Most importantly I would like to start by thanking my wife, son, parents, and brothers for their unconditional love, kindness, and patience.

I would like to thank the following friends for their energy, inspiration, and guidance throughout this project: Ana Matos, Brad Hults, Dave Cormier, Dawnmarie McIntosh, Shannon and Dan Smith, David Yeh, Yvonne Heyne, Karen Williams, Toni Brodelle, Marcel Hutten, Becky Blake, Dillon Dhanecha, Karl Whitfield, John and Christina Amaral, Laurence Blume, Doug Allen, and Loren Slocum, for writing such a generous foreword.

Special thanks to Tony, Sage, and everyone within the Platinum Family and also to Mitch, Sheila, Elise, Eland, Helen, Kirby, Katie, and everyone within the Advantage Family.

Finally, I would like to acknowledge and thank you for showing a greater interest in your health and well-being. I truly hope you find what you are looking for amongst these pages.

To your health . . .

# ABOUT THE AUTHOR

Dr. Shan Hussain is a general practitioner working in partnership at a large family practice near his hometown of Nottingham, England. He graduated from Imperial College School of Medicine, London, in 1999. Since completing his postgraduate training and joining his partnership in 2007, he has developed a keen interest in the promotion of health and well-being. He has also studied coaching, neuro-linguistic programming, and is currently working on a PhD in psychoneurology. In addition to practising health care, he enjoys reading, music, forex trading, culinary arts, travel, and adventure with family and friends.

*"The doctor of the future will give no medicine, but will interest patients in care of the human frame, in diet, and in the cause and prevention of disease."*

**—Thomas Edison**

# INTRODUCTION

It was the end of the busiest Monday morning of my life. I felt exhausted after completing more than forty consultations, with each patient describing an average of two problems they wanted me to fix. It was a great relief that I had fifteen minutes to spare before my next clinical commitment, but little consolation that thousands of doctors across the country had experienced a similar morning.

As I took a few deep breaths to rest my mind and allow my thoughts to settle, I found myself wondering how many of today's patients could have avoided seeing a doctor this morning. I reflected on the list of people I had seen and individually reviewed my notes for each of them. How many of these illnesses were preventable? Are these prevention strategies widely available? How often are they adopted?

I found myself getting into dangerous territory. It was clear that many of today's patients had presented problems associated with adopted lifestyles. However, I felt that conveying this message to patients may not necessarily be greeted well. Some may incorrectly accuse me of blaming them for their problems, not realising how deeply I care for their health. But it's certainly very convenient to think that some illnesses just "happen" and a pill will fix it all.

I began to reflect on the concept of responsibility. Who is truly responsible for the long-term health of patients? Is it the doctor, or the patient, or both of us? Does my role as a doctor really shift absolute responsibility of someone's long-term health entirely onto my shoulders forever?

The truth is that doctors can do their very best to treat illness, but if the cause of illness is due to the patient's adopted lifestyle choices coupled with a reluctance to change, then the illness is unlikely to ever be cured—at best, it will be "clinically managed."

Clinical management covers a wide variety of interventions, including surgery, medications, and counselling, and the chosen intervention depends on the condition involved. For example, an inflamed, ruptured appendix obviously needs urgent surgical removal and no other intervention is yet proven to be successful.

However, I believe that many conditions such as type 2 diabetes or hypertension (raised blood pressure) are commonly treated with medication before all other avenues have truly been exhausted. Many people who take prescribed medication to treat hypertension could have their blood pressure controlled if they were to stop smoking, lose excessive weight, exercise, optimise their diet, and reduce stress. This five-step formula alone could save the health-care system billions of pounds every year, but unfortunately it is not fully applied. I feel this is not because of ignorance but perceived difficulties in application. People find themselves getting overwhelmed by asking themselves, "How can I possibly do that?" or worse still, "Why should I bother with that when I can just take a few pills?" This is an area that I will explore fully later in this book.

I believe that the only sustainable model to long-term health care is one where patients and doctors align and collaborate to help reach the individuals' desired health goals. Unless we truly work together, neither of our goals will be achieved. This is where the future of health care should lie.

The World Health Organization defines health as "a state of complete physical, mental, and social well being and not merely the absence of disease or infirmity."[1] This powerful statement was written into the WHO Constitution on 7 April 1948, and to this day has never been amended.

I remember first hearing this definition as a young medical student more than twenty years ago in a crowded lecture hall at my university in London. As I looked around the room packed with 120 fellow students, I wondered to myself, *How many people in here can really say they are healthy? In fact, can anyone truly say they are healthy?*

I have often reflected on this definition over the years.

*Complete* physical well-being.

*Complete* mental well-being.

*Complete* social well-being.

What does this look like?

How do we quantify it?

And how much can doctors really do to help people achieve such high levels of well-being?

I believe that focussing on the three areas of physical, mental, and social well-being and working to improve each one individually is by definition the key to achieving better health. An individual may have good mental health and physical health, but if their social health is neglected, this can lead to an imbalance and possibly illness, as I will describe later. Poor physical or mental well-being will also impact the other areas—ideally, all three should be in balance.

---

1   "WHO definition of health," World Health Organization, http://www.who.int/about/definition/en/print.html.

In my experience, many doctors in the 21st century are analogous to firefighters—constantly responding to emergencies. But in actual fact, firefighters do not save nearly as many lives as fire-safety officers—the prevention of fire is what really saves lives. Hence, the old adage from Erasmus: "Prevention is better than cure."

I feel that doctors should also take this approach to a greater level. Teaching men and women about health and well-being helps to save lives. Preventing a disease from happening in the first place is much easier than treating it after it has taken hold. So many of the diseases I see every day are somewhat preventable: type 2 diabetes, high blood pressure, obesity, heart disease, stroke, even some cancers. How? By making small simple lifestyle changes that have a compounding effect over time to help a patient reach their health goals.

It is for this reason that I have written this book. I hope to help you understand the many ways that illnesses may arise and also show you how positive lifestyle choices can not only help prevent these illnesses from developing but also improve levels of health, well-being, energy, and vitality.

It is my great pleasure to guide you through the information in this book and help you to identify areas in your life that may adversely impact long-term health and well-being. If you find the information has been helpful or not, I would welcome your feedback.

# CHAPTER 1

# THE FOUNDATIONS OF HEALTH

What is health? How would you personally define health? And what would better health mean for you?

We all have different images of health. Some relate health to their physical appearance or their energy levels, or simply how they feel in themselves. Others equate health to just having the ability to survive the day.

I would like you to take a moment to consider the World Health Organization's definition of health: "a state of complete physical, mental, and social well-being."

What would this level of health feel like for you? How would it improve your energy levels, your appearance, your relationships with close ones, your job, your income, your confidence, your self-image, your social standing, or your future?

With this in mind, I would like to start by inviting you to write down a list of your top five reasons why you personally want better health and what it would mean for you.

1.

2.

3.

4.

5.

Your vision of good health begins by paying attention to and taking care of every aspect of yourself. I encourage you to start thinking about health from three perspectives:

- physical health (the body)

- mental health (the mind)

- social health (interactions with the environment)

In the simplest of terms, when these three components are fully nurtured, we move towards health. When they are ignored, neglected, or not fully addressed, we move towards disease.

Again, to keep things simple, consider the following principles:

1. What we put into and what we eliminate from our physical body will help determine the state of our physical health.

2. Thoughts, feelings, and emotions—and how we manage these—will help determine our mental health.

3. How (and who) we interact within our environment will help determine our social health.

## YOU ARE WHAT YOU CONSUME

The great French epicure Jean Anthelme Brillat-Savarin stated, "Tell me what you eat, and I will tell you what you are." That was back in the early 1800s, but his observation is still valid. I believe that you are not only what you eat but also what you absorb and assimilate from your environment.

We are what we eat on a constitutional level, but I believe who you are is also related to what else you consume. What are you absorbing? What are you reading? What are you watching? Who are you spending time with? What experiences are you having? All these elements can get absorbed into the mind, on a conscious or subconscious level. You are what you absorb, on every level. This has an impact who you are as a person, how you behave, how you act, and how you interact with others.

If we change our consumption habits, then we can change who we are. Look at what you eat and drink, but also look at everything else you're absorbing from your environment. This may include social media, television, magazines, books, movies, and also the people you spend most time with. Find the right balance that supports your health.

## HEALTH AND RESPONSIBILITY

The last thing I want to do is make people think, *My disease is all my fault*. It's not about fault. Casting blame doesn't solve the problem; rather, positive change comes about by recognising the problem and making adjustments that can combat its ill effects. It's not about taking blame; it's about taking greater care and responsibility. If you see your health as something you can take greater ownership of, then you can be empowered to do something about it. But if you see a disease as your "fault," then you're immediately starting from a negative place.

We will soon describe many healthy lifestyle choices one can make, but I don't usually recommend making several big changes immediately after recognising a health problem, simply because wholesale changes may not be easy to sustain. You'll do a lot more to help yourself if you gradually introduce sustainable changes into your daily routine.

Take note when things are going well, and don't reproach yourself when they aren't. It's better to just recognise that your approach isn't working and ask yourself why. Once you understand why an attempted change isn't working, you'll be able to adjust your approach. There are many different ways to improve your health, and some will work better for you than others.

I firmly believe that one of my roles as a doctor is not to pass judgment. Rather, my role is to help patients take control of their health by providing the information they need to make choices that support their health goals, whether that be losing weight, controlling blood pressure, or simply feeling healthier and more energised.

It's also vital to set realistic goals. For example, if you're fifty pounds overweight and say to yourself, "I'll lose fifty pounds over the next year," that can be done. Losing one or two pounds a week is an achievable goal. Not only that—losing this weight can be done in a healthy manner and, most importantly, in an enjoyable way.

## ENJOY THE JOURNEY

Finding ways to enjoy a healthy lifestyle can motivate you to take control of your health. This truth became more apparent for me personally while I was recently visiting with some old friends. I remember one of them had lost a tremendous amount of weight and was in very impressive physical shape. The rest of us were shocked at his transformation.

I told my friend that the years had been kind to him and asked him what he'd been doing to lose weight and stay in such great shape. He told us he had simply been exercising every day and just looking after himself. I asked how he kept himself motivated, as I found exercise to be rather dull, and I noticed he became a little guarded. Eventually, he told us that when he goes to the gym every day, he constantly plays the training montage from a famous boxing movie on his iPod. We all started laughing until he stood up and lifted his shirt and showed us his abs. At that point, the laughter stopped pretty quickly.

This encounter with my friend showed me that whatever works for you is just fine, as long is it isn't harmful. If certain music inspires you to go to the gym more regularly, then it doesn't matter if your old friends find that funny. Let them laugh.

My friend found a way to make his time at the gym enjoyable, and he stuck to it. He had a goal, he committed to it, and he found a way to keep up his routine every single day for just thirty minutes. His mantra when he wakes up in the morning is, "I'm not getting back in this bed until I've been to the gym. My day is not complete until I've exercised." That is his rule, and he never breaks it, which is how he achieved the results.

## PREVENTABLE ILLNESSES

As mentioned earlier, many chronic illnesses are largely preventable through better diet and lifestyle. Obesity and type 2 diabetes are near the top of the list, but really, most nongenetic illnesses can potentially be avoided or delayed. Many such illnesses fall under the same umbrella simply because they reflect an imbalance in an individual's physical, mental, or social well-being. Therefore the approach to helping prevent them is essentially the same. Prevention is about taking care of and improving your physical, mental, and social health. If there is a significant imbalance in any of those three things, that imbalance can manifest as disease. Of course, we're all a little different. If I have the same imbalance as you, that doesn't necessarily mean it would manifest as the same disease for both of us.

It has been shown by the National Heart, Lung, and Blood Institute that being overweight or obese increases your risk of developing type 2 diabetes, heart disease, hypertension, stroke, and osteoarthritis, as well as some cancers, such as breast cancer and bowel cancer.[2] Those are seven illnesses with preventable elements to them. And among those seven, there is a significant amount of overlap. I have not met many patients who are obese and who don't also have type 2 diabetes. Similarly, I have not met many patients who have heart disease and don't also have hypertension.

## THE ROLE OF STRESS

The word *stress* gets used pretty loosely and frequently—something that is just mildly annoying often gets called *stressful*. As a doctor, I regard stress as any physical, mental, or emotional factor that causes strain or tension to the body or mind. Mental or emotional stress often results from adverse situations, such as family conflict, worries about work, or health issues, but it's important to remember that stress is highly individual. What's highly stressful for one person may be regarded as normal for another. Whenever a patient tells me they feel ill or mentally exhausted or depressed from stress, I take it seriously, even if the stress they describe doesn't seem all that stressful. After all, I believe physical, mental, or social stress may well be the fundamental basis of most, if not all, disease.

The fact that stress is so variable among individuals suggests that stress has subjective elements to it. It's what we *perceive* as stressful and how we *react* to that perception that leads to feeling stressed.

2    "What Are the Health Risks of Overweight and Obesity?" National Heart, Lung, and Blood Institute, www.nhlbi.nih.gov/health/health-topics/topics/obe/risks.

Unfortunately, stress has a real physiological effect on the body. Stress has a huge impact on your biochemistry and hormones. It not only increases your heart rate and blood pressure but can also trigger many different behaviour patterns as well. When we're stressed, some people turn to the fridge and eat everything in there. Others may react to stress by having a cigarette. Some sit in front of the television with an alcoholic beverage. What all these examples have in common is that individuals are seeking some sort of distraction to escape from stress.

It may be helpful to recognise the role that the individual's perception plays in processing stress. Are they experiencing something that is truly stressful, like a family bereavement or losing a job, or is it something that is simply perceived as stressful? Would it be possible to regard the situation differently?

I don't know when stress became a medical diagnosis, but on a typical day in practise I might see five patients who describe stress as their problem. When we talk about what's causing the stress, they'll usually describe a professional, personal, relationship, or financial problem—sometimes a combination of all.

Displacing their stress onto the body may cause people to experience many different symptoms, such as chronic headaches, irritable bowel symptoms, skin eruptions, or feeling tired all the time. Stress is also recognised as a contributory factor to several medical conditions including obesity, heart disease, Alzheimer's disease, type 2 diabetes, depression, anxiety, gastric ulcers, inflammatory bowel disease, and asthma.

## CHANGING THE PERCEPTION

A few years ago while I felt I was going through a really stressful time, I remember catching up with an old friend after work. After we exchanged pleasantries, I shared how much stress I had been under, without going into any detail. His reaction surprised me, "I'll tell you the real reason you're stressed—you've said yes to things that you should have said no to."

He went on, "Right now, you're choosing to be stressed subconsciously. Maybe you need to make some better choices."

That certainly gave me something to reflect on. How much of our stress is real? How much is just a perception? How much stress are we inviting into our lives without knowing it?

I realised that whilst I had so much on my plate at the time, it was me who had put many of those things on the plate. Nobody else put them there. So I was left with two choices: take some things off my plate, or get a bigger plate!

If you find yourself feeling you have too much on your plate, consider regarding your tasks differently. You might feel that you're being forced to do things, but you're often really not.

The truth is that you don't have to do anything you don't want to do. There may be consequences to your inactions, but you always have choices. You have free will if you live in a free society. Look at things that you perhaps are devoting too much time and attention to. What can you delegate? What can wait? What is important right now and what isn't? What is causing unnecessary stress right now? What can you let go of right now?

We all like to help people however we can. We want to say yes. We want to make people happy and help them to meet their needs. But if you are overextended and harming your own health as a result, then the truth is you're helping no one.

## TIME-OUT

In the UK, we hear a lot of unfair media reports about a so-called "sick-note culture." People go to their doctors feigning illness to get a medical certificate to sign them off work. However, there is an opposite problem of greater proportion that gets very little attention: people who refuse sick notes. They refuse to take time off work because they are so loyal to their organisation. They don't want to let anyone down—or they fear losing their job if they seem to be less committed. They're scared. They're fearful. They feel a strong obligation to go into work, even if they're running a high fever, vomiting every hour, and dizzy. They will still go to work, displacing even more stress on their body.

When I tell my patients to not return to work—to allow the body the time it needs to recover—some initially reject this advice, fearing what they will get behind on at work. I emphasise that no amount of work is worth risking their health and the health of others at the workplace. The body needs time to recover, to rest, to heal. Healing can only take place by giving the body what it needs to return to a healthy state—and a sick body needs rest.

## THE REST YOU NEED

Many people in our society don't often get the rest they need. A lot of us are in a "sleep debt." We try to make it up on the weekends by having a lie-in, but that doesn't usually work. If you have children, a lie-in only lasts a short while, until 7:30 a.m....if you are lucky. Catching up on sleep, going to bed a little earlier, and giving your body the physical rest it needs does wonders for your constitution. Sleep can help you be so much more effective the next day at work. This important area will be covered in more detail later.

Along with the rest, you must participate in the physical activity that lets your body want the rest. After all, we live in cycles of activity and rest. The more active we are, mentally and physically, the more rest we get. Certainly if you've had an active day, you're more likely to fall asleep easily. And a mentally active day can be just as exhausting as a physically active day.

## EXERCISE: JUST DO IT

*"Lack of activity destroys the good condition of every human being, while movement and methodical physical exercise save it and preserve it."*

### —Plato

Exercise is proven beyond doubt to be beneficial in the prevention and treatment of so many conditions, including cardiovascular disease, diabetes, depression, and even some cancers.[3]

A 2014 study showed that people who regularly go for a run can reduce their chances of dying from a cardiovascular cause by 55 per cent and also reduce their all-cause mortality by 30 per cent—even if running for just one hour a week.[4] If there were a pill that could reduce chances of dying by 30 per cent, wouldn't most of us want it?

Making small, simple, sustained changes in your life can yield huge changes in your health, but it's important to plan realistically. If

3    Peter Kokkinos, "Physical Activity, Health Benefits, and Mortality Risk," ISRN Cardiology, 2012 (2012), http://dx.doi.org/10.5402/2012/718789.

4    Duck-chul Lee, Russell R. Pate, Carl J. Lavie, Sui Xuemei, Timothy S. Church, Steven N. Blair, "Leisure-Time Running Reduces All-Cause and Cardiovascular Mortality Risk," Journal of the American College of Cardiology, 64 (2014): 472–481, doi:10.1016/j.jacc.2014.04.058.

you're overweight and decide you're only going to eat one thousand calories a day, that's not going to work. It won't work because one thousand calories a day is not enough to sustain the average human being. You'll feel tired and sluggish and crave sugar. You'll be off that diet quickly. Cutting out your daily sugary coffee with whipped cream, however, would help you eliminate calories and move towards a healthier diet.

The same is true for exercise. If you don't regularly exercise, deciding to work out for an hour a day isn't going to get you onto a regular exercise schedule—you'll feel terrible from overexerting yourself, and you won't be eager to get back to the gym. You might even suffer an injury. It's far better to start with a gentle exercise program of just fifteen minutes daily and add ten minutes more each week. Stop when you reach an hour. Working out longer than that probably won't be increasingly beneficial.

Just start easy. Start light. Start fun. Ensure you're enjoying whatever form of exercise you choose. If an activity is hurting or if you don't want to do it, don't do it. Find something that works better for you. Most importantly—just start.

If you don't know where to start, go to a gym. Gyms are stocked with tools and equipment, along with people who can help you use them and give advice and recommendations that can help you reach your physical goals.

Building up momentum is important. Yes, you're making a needed change, but you still may need to talk yourself into it. If you say aloud, "I'm going to go to the gym right now. I'm now putting on my trainers. I'm putting on my exercise clothing. I'm physically walking out the door," then your brain will eventually catch up!

I remember hearing the renowned coach Tony Robbins once say, "How many times have you sat down and said, 'I'm just going to sit down for two minutes' and before you know it, half an hour has passed?" He recommended applying this same principle to exercise, and I often share this suggestion with my patients. Coach yourself—*I'm going to pedal on this exercise bike only for thirty seconds.* And once you have pushed past that first thirty seconds, you'll begin to build up that time. *Just five more minutes . . .* Before you know it, you'll do that five minutes easily, and then maybe feel you could go on for ten or maybe fifteen minutes.

Trainers often advise their clients to participate in an activity for five minutes and to stop, if they want, after that initial period. Once they have gathered momentum, they are less likely to want to stop.

When I studied physics at school, our first lesson was about overcoming inertia. If you imagine there is a block of wood on a table and you want to shift that block slightly to the right, the force required to get that movement started is much more than the force needed to keep it moving steadily after that. That initial movement is called the *limiting static friction force*, which requires more energy than the *momentum force*. Once it's moving, a lot less force is needed to keep it moving. The same principal applies with exercise. Overcome that inertia, and you can keep going.

If you build up that momentum, you won't have to force yourself to the gym. The first trip is the toughest. Once you create the time to start doing it and you get yourself in the habit, it's a lot easier. If you can surround yourself with and befriend a peer group of exercisers, then that can greatly increase your incentive to want to get to the gym. If a like-minded group of people coax you to meet them at the gym at 7:00 a.m., you'll be there because you don't want to disappoint them and because their company is enjoyable. They make your workout more exciting. After a surprisingly short time, your gym visits become easier. Eventually, you look forward to them. You then miss exercising if you don't do it.

So just start. Start right now if you can. Don't give your brain time to talk yourself out of it. If you can't start immediately, at least head to an online store now and purchase a good quality rebounder or mini trampoline. I will explain why I value these so highly in chapter 3.

# CHAPTER 2

# PHYSICAL HEALTH

*"If we could give every individual the right amount of nourishment and exercise, not too little and not too much, we would have found the safest way to health."*

**—Hippocrates**

## PHYSICAL HEALTH: THE BODY

It is a popular scientific belief in some quarters that our bodies fully regenerate themselves every seven years. This means that, at a constitutional level, you are not the same physical person that you were seven years ago. Personally, I am uncertain about this seven-year theory. However, I cannot ignore the powerful capacity that our bodies have to regenerate. Each of our estimated forty trillion cells has a limited life span before it dies and is replaced. For example, the average life span of our red blood cells is four months. Our skin regenerates every two to four weeks. Our liver regenerates every five months.

Our bodies get the raw materials they require to regenerate from our diet. There are only eight essential components of a healthy diet:

1. Water

2. Proteins

3. Fats

4. Carbohydrates

5. Vitamins

6. Minerals

7. Fibre

8. Oxygen

We need an adequate intake of all these components every single day. Unfortunately, despite a lot of research, we still don't know exactly how much of each component is needed. What is clearer, however, is the fact that an imbalance of our intake of any of these components can cause illness. For example, inadequate water intake can lead to dehydration, lethargy, headaches, skin conditions, and kidney problems, amongst many others. Excessive carbohydrates can lead to weight gain or type 2 diabetes. Inadequate fibre can lead to digestive problems. The list goes on.

Start to think of the physical body as a system that is constantly regenerating. We need to take in the correct raw materials to allow this regeneration, but at the same time, we need to allow the body to eliminate the waste material we create from our cells' activities and turnover.

How do we encourage this elimination? There are four main elimination channels:

1. Lungs

2. Skin

3. Bowels

4. Urinary tract

What happens when we are unable to eliminate the waste we build up through one of these channels? Obviously, we end up carrying this waste material around, which may later manifest as disease.

## THE PHYSICAL BODY IN CONSTANT REGENERATION

**INPUT**

1.  WATER
2.  PROTEINS
3.  FATS
4.  CARBOHYDRATES
5.  VITAMINS
6.  MINERALS
7.  FIBRE
8.  OXYGEN

**OUTPUT**

ELIMINATION OF WASTE THROUGH:

1.  LUNGS
2.  SKIN
3.  BOWELS
4.  URINARY TRACT

To support this constant regeneration, it is important to ensure that we have a healthy intake of good quality air and nutrients (which I will discuss later under NORMAL foods) and also encourage and support all four of these elimination channels.

## DIETARY CHANGES

**Drink water.** The first dietary change I recommend has nothing to do with food. Start drinking water instead of any and all other beverages. Drink plain water, maybe with a squeeze of lemon juice for additional flavour, vitamins, and minerals. Most store-bought drinks aren't good for you, although I do recommend (in moderation) fresh homemade vegetable and fruit juices made with a quality juicer.

If you truly want to restore, maintain, and sustain your health, firstly look at your fluid intake. While there may be good things (such as antioxidants) in coffee, you don't assimilate the water in coffee particularly well. The caffeine in coffee is a diuretic that causes you to pass more urine. Drinking coffee may even cause you to lose more water than the amount of water you're consuming from the coffee itself.

We lose around three to four litres of water every day through our sweat, exhaled air, bowel movements, and urination. Some of this water is created as a by-product of metabolic processes. As much as one to two litres of water are lost every single day just by breathing.

We have to replace most of the water we lose, and there is no better way to do that than by simply consuming water. Whilst there is water contained in most of the food we eat, the average person still needs to drink around two to three litres of water every day. I've seen many patients benefit hugely just from drinking more water. Water has tremendous impacts on health in terms of weight loss, skin hydration, and energy levels. You can change your health for the better simply by drinking more water.

A recent study suggested that people sometimes mistake thirst for hunger.[5] You think you're feeling hungry, so you eat something, but what your body really wants is water, not food. Eating doesn't solve the underlying problem, but it often causes weight gain. In the meantime, you're still not getting the fluid you need, so you feel tired and sluggish. To get over that, you may end up drinking something with caffeine in it and lose even more fluid. The next time you feel tired and think you need a coffee, try drinking a large glass of water and take some deep breaths instead. You'll probably feel more alert than if you drank the coffee.

In moderation, freshly squeezed fruit and vegetable juices from a quality home juicer are a good alternative to water. They must be fresh, with nothing added. That way, you know that you're getting just the juice itself. Fresh juice has not been through any pasteurization process or artificial process to change the actual constituency of the natural goodness. It doesn't have any added sugar.

Fresh homemade juice is a lightning quick way to get nutrients into your body. It puts little stress on the digestive system, and some of the nutrients are absorbed immediately from the tongue and the mouth. Juice can actually can give you an energy boost, which, in my experience, is as good as or better than caffeine. It's the body saying, *Right, this is what I wanted.* I highly recommend drinking fresh juice daily, preferably from a masticating juicer, as they retain more fibre and the juice will stay fresh longer.

---

5    F. McKiernan, J.H. Hollis, G McCabe, and R.D. Mattes, "Thirst-drinking, hunger-eating; tight coupling?", *J Am Diet Assoc.*, 109 (2009): 486–490, doi: 10.1016/j.jada.2008.11.027.

## NORMAL FOOD

*"Let food be your medicine and medicine be your food."*

### —Hippocrates

What you eat and drink is central to getting and staying healthy. If you truly want to get the quality of nutrients your body needs to sustain and repair itself, I recommend focusing on NORMAL foods:

Natural

Organic

Raw

Meat-free

Additive-free

Lactose- and dairy-free

**Natural.** A fresh apple is logically going to be a lot better for you than an apple pie. We want to eat foods in their natural form, not as part of highly refined, manufactured, or processed systems. Processing removes much of foods' natural goodness and nutrients, while adding sugar, salt, and unnatural chemicals. As I tell my patients, you can't go too far wrong by eating fresh vegetables, fruits, and salads.

**Organic.** Natural eating aligns you more with real food. Organic foods are grown without the use of artificial fertilizers and pesticides.

Animal products are raised without added hormones or antibiotics and under more humane conditions. Are organic foods really any better for you than their less expensive, conventionally produced alternatives? Well, there are many conflicting studies and the jury remains out, but whilst we await the verdict, I have a simple question: Do you want the toxic residues of the many, many chemicals used in conventionally produced food in your body? We don't know the long-term effects of these toxins. We don't know the damage that they are potentially doing to us already. What we do know is that these chemicals are dangerous if they're consumed on their own. Why are we consuming them with our food? Let's have some common sense about this and avoid them. Have your food without them—stick to organic.

**Raw.** Eat your fruits and vegetables raw and fresh whenever possible and appropriate, simply because this preserves the most nutrients. Eating a raw carrot is always going to be better than eating a micro-waved carrot or a baked carrot with brown sugar, or even consuming fresh carrot juice. A lot of the internal goodness remains and is most easily digestible if you haven't denatured it through cooking or processing. The next best alternative to raw is to steam vegetables, as this form of cooking will still preserve many nutrients.

**Meat-Free.** I'm not promoting vegetarianism, but I recognise that balance is key. Meat, unfortunately, has a lot of things in it that aren't so good for us, including saturated fat. Diets high in meat have been linked to many diseases, such as bowel cancer. Many people don't want to give up meat forever. There's no reason to eliminate it from your diet completely, unless you have personal or moral reasons for doing so. I recommend aiming for eighty/twenty. Aim to avoid meat in 80 per cent of your meals if you don't wish to eliminate it altogether from your diet.

**Additive-Free.** Avoiding additives in your food is an extension of eating organic. If you eat organic foods whenever possible, you reduce the amount of added chemicals, such as preservatives and salt, that may be in your food. Many processed foods, even those that are made with organic ingredients, still may have a lot of additives. Why does a natural food need additives? Natural foods were eaten without additives for thousands of years. Many additives are preservatives that make the food last longer before it gets mouldy, stale, or otherwise goes bad. Do you really want these substances in your body? Beyond convenience, I see no evidence of the positive impact of food additives on the health of the population.

**Lactose- and Dairy-Free.** Many people don't have the ability to digest lactose, the sugar found in milk and dairy products such as yogurt. I see this with some of my patients. Many patients who come to me describing digestive problems turn out to be lactose-intolerant. Their body doesn't produce the enzyme to digest lactose. They may get stomach cramps, gas, bloating, and/or diarrhoea from dairy. Giving up these foods often clears up digestive problems.

I can share many anecdotes of patients with allergies, asthma, and skin conditions such as eczema and psoriasis that have been cured simply by eliminating dairy.

When I tell this to people, they almost always object that if you don't drink milk or eat dairy foods, then you won't get enough calcium. The opposite is actually true. The calcium from dairy foods is not absorbed well and does not contribute to bone health. Dr Amy

Lanou, PhD, nutrition director for the Physicians Committee for Responsible Medicine in Washington, D.C., has studied this area closely and concluded the following: "The countries with the highest rates of osteoporosis are the ones where people drink the most milk… and the connection between dairy consumption and bone health is almost nonexistent."[6]

The healthier and more natural way to get dietary calcium is by eating green leafy vegetables, such as kale and broccoli. Good alternatives to cow's milk are almond milk and coconut milk.

I recommend eating NORMAL foods at least 80 per cent of the time. The goal here is not to take things away from you or make you feel deprived. Nor is it about telling you what to do or judging you if you don't do it. It's about striking a sensible balance that will help support your physical health. If you want to have cheese and don't want to eliminate it from your diet, incorporate it moderately. Just be aware of the drawbacks and try to balance your diet with other, healthier foods. If you eat a healthier diet 80 per cent of the time, or even 50 per cent of the time, then you've made a great start. You've done yourself a huge favour by changing your diet for the better. Start with changes that are simple and achievable. Every time you put good nourishment into your body, you're moving forward.

Eating a more NORMAL diet requires reduction (or even elimination) of foods that are not NORMAL. These "non-NORMAL" foods include processed foods, especially those rich in sugar or starch such as cake, chips, and other snacks. Non-NORMAL foods also include the six white foods that I recommend avoiding: flour, sugar, rice, pasta, potatoes, and salt. Starchy foods such as breads, pasta, and potatoes are converted to glucose, or blood sugar, quickly. When

---

6   Vivian Goldschmidt, MA, "Debunking the Milk Myth: Why Milk Is Bad for You and Your Bones," Save Institute, http://saveourbones.com/osteoporosis-milk-myth/.

you eat them, your pancreas produces extra insulin, the hormone that carries blood sugar into your cells to be used for energy or stored as fat. A diet high in these foods has been associated with obesity, elevated blood-sugar levels, and type 2 diabetes.

These white foods are also mostly low in fibre and associated with irritable bowel syndrome and bloating. You may get the perception that you're full, when in reality you're just bloated. It's important to understand that distinction. You're not going to feel full until you've truly consumed the nutrients that your body is craving.

I once had a patient who said he'd tried "everything" to lose weight. I suggested he eliminated the six white foods and dairy products. Two weeks later, he made an emergency appointment to see me. I worried something had happened to him.

When the patient came in and sat down, he blurted out, "I just wanted to tell you that I've lost 7 lbs in the past two weeks."

I said, "Great, what's the emergency?"

"Oh, no emergency. I'm just so excited and really wanted to tell that to you!"

I can't say that was the best use of an emergency clinic, but I was obviously very happy with this positive news and his results and encouraged him to keep going.

## KEEPING IT OFF

The sad truth is that many people who lose excessive weight regain at least some of it. Keeping weight off is difficult if you view losing weight as a process that ends when you reach your goal. It's more a process of permanently changing your approach to what you eat and taking greater care of yourself. If you overexercise or starve yourself to lose weight, then you'll almost certainly regain it.

The better approach is to evaluate what standards you are holding yourself to. Could you set a better standard to support your health and well-being? Would keeping your weight healthy boost your energy, strength, confidence, and self-esteem?

I encourage people who want to lose weight to first imagine what would happen if they lost their excess weight. What would that mean to them? How great would that be? How much better would they look? Would they be able to get back into their favourite jeans? When they have more energy and feel better about themselves, will their career prospects improve? I ask them to create a clear vision for what they want to achieve. Creating a compelling image of a better version of themselves helps them to build the stamina necessary to stick with weight-loss activities.

In my experience, the people who lose weight and keep it off have really defined *why* weight loss is important to them. They have clear and compelling reasons for wanting to lose weight. They shift their standards. Once they get to their target, they feel better about themselves. That feeling is addictive. It's a feeling of accomplishment, achievement, confidence, power, and so much more.

## ELIMINATION

Eliminating waste from your body efficiently is a much bigger factor in maintaining good health than people realize. There are four elimination channels: the skin, lungs, bowels, and urinary tract. It is vital to promote and support elimination from all four of these channels. Efficient elimination will increase how quickly we release toxins and wastes from our body, and this can also give an energy boost and help prevent disease.

**Breathing Exercises**. To improve elimination of waste carbon dioxide through the lungs, I recommend deep-breathing exercises.

When people are stressed or anxious, one of the first things they do is stop breathing effectively by taking shorter and shallower breaths.

I recommend taking deep, regular breaths from the diaphragm. Try this exercise now: place your palms flat on your stomach, with your index fingertips touching each other, and your middle fingertips also touching each other, making a little diamond around your navel. As you take a deep breath in, your fingertips will be pulled apart, making your stomach look "fat". The more they part, the better you're breathing from your diaphragm. And when you exhale, exhale completely, as far as you can. I recommend doing this exercise five to ten times in one go and repeating it two or three times a day. Just inhale, hold, exhale, and repeat. It gets more oxygen into your blood-stream by increasing your lung capacity as much as 30 per cent, and its also helps with lymphatic drainage. Some people like to inhale, hold, and then exhale for varying counts. Do what's comfortable. As long as you're getting the increased oxygen into your body and you're breathing from the diaphragm, then you'll get the result you need. Try it now.

If you're feeling tired for no obvious reason, it could well be because you haven't been breathing correctly for a while. The trick I use when I feel tired is to breathe deeply, holding each breath for a few seconds at the deepest part of the inhalation. Then I breathe out and let my diaphragm drop passively as far as it wants to. Doing this exercise for only a few minutes is a great energy booster and can also help during times of heightened stress.

**Hydration.** To improve elimination through the urinary tract, drinking more water is helpful. You'll start to pass more urine, and you'll know you're drinking enough when your urine is clear and colourless. If your urine has any colour to it, then chances are you may be somewhat dehydrated. When the urine is colourless, you know that your fluid intake is, in fact, flushing out your system properly.

**Fibre.** Elimination through the bowel is a bit more complicated. In medical school, we were taught that normal bowel movements happen anywhere from three times a day to every three days. Personally, I feel if you're going anything less than once daily, then you've built up a backlog of faecal matter that needs clearing out. It should be done naturally through increasing fibre in the diet. It's crucial to also increase water intake and activity. In fact, when my patients start drinking more water, they tell me their sluggish bowels also start moving better.

Fibre is found in all plant-based foods and is regarded as an essential component of our diets, but the body does not absorb it. Nonetheless, there have been numerous studies showing the benefits of high-fibre diets. A recent showed that a high-fibre diet (35 g per day) lowered the risk of dying from cardiovascular disease by as much as 54 per cent and also lowered the risk of death from *all causes* by 37 per cent.[7]

The right amount of fibre may vary from person to person. What's important is getting a sensible amount of it with every meal. Another contributory factor to constipation is a lack of physical activity, and many studies have shown the benefits of exercise in preventing constipation as well as other bowel conditions such as colon cancer, diverticular disease, and gallstones.

Often, people are slightly constipated without realizing it. They may feel a bit off or sluggish. When they improve their fibre intake

---

7    P. Buil-Cosiales, I. Zazpe, E. Toledo, D. Corella, J. Salas-Salvadó, J. Diez-Espino, E. Ros, J. Fernandez-Creuet Navajas, J. Manuel Santos-Lozano, F. Arós, M. Fiol, O. Castañer, L. Serra-Majem, X. Pintó, R. Lamuela-Raventós, A. Marti, F. Basterra-Gortari, J. Sorlí, J. Verdú-Rotellar, J. Basora, V. Ruiz-Gutierrez, R. Estruch, and M. Martínez-González, "Fiber intake and all-cause mortality in the Prevención con Dieta Meditrerránea (PREDIMED) study," *American Journal of Clinical Nutrition*, 2014, doi: 10.3945/ajcn.114.093757.

and add more water for other reasons, such as weight loss, they often find that their bowels improve, and they feel a lot better.

However, if you notice a significant change in your bowel habits, particular if they are looser for no reason and there is blood or mucus in your motions, it is vital that you seek urgent medical advice.

I've found that constipation is becoming a real problem with children who often end up eating a lot of processed food low in fibre and don't drink enough water or get enough exercise. The child might have obvious symptoms, such as bloating and abdominal pain. Chronic constipation can also make a child feel tired or cranky and can even lead to behavioural issues. Therefore, addressing constipation in children is of the utmost importance.

Bowel problems can also be related to stress and emotions, making things move too quickly or too slowly. Look at all bowel issues holistically—what else is going on to cause a change in bowel habits? We focus on fluids, fibre, exercise, and then address any emotional imbalance that might be contributing.

**Skin.** The final elimination channel is the skin. Your skin is actually your largest organ. It's the protective barrier between you and the environment. When you sweat, you regulate your body's temperature and also eliminate toxins and excess salt. You also shed thousands of dead skin cells every minute, which stimulates the growth of fresh new cells.

It is, therefore, vital to make sure to preserve the heath of your skin and to encourage this elimination channel. Having a good balanced diet with sufficient water intake certainly helps, as does exercise, which encourages perspiration. To help promote this elimination channel, Ayurvedic medicine has long practised gentle skin brushing (exfoliation) with a simple dry skin brush. The theory behind this is that it helps clear clogged pores in the skin that inhibit effective sweating, whilst also brushing away skin cells and surface toxins and stimulating the lymphatic system. To encourage sweating, I also recommend spending some time in a sauna. A recent study in the *Journal of the American Medical Association* showed that regular use of a sauna can reduce your chances of developing cardiovascular disease and help you live longer. The heat causes you to sweat out accumulated toxins and waste products and also improve your circulation. Nonetheless, please seek appropriate medical advice before regular use of a sauna.[8]

## WHAT NOT TO DRINK

*"Don't consume anything with an ingredients label!"*

**—Dr Frank Shallenberger**

If you're serious about getting your health back in balance, I suggest avoiding energy drinks and alcohol.

Before you down that energy drink to get over being tired or having a hangover, look at the ingredients on the label. Other than water, the mixture of ingredients rarely, if ever, contains anything natural. If there's something you don't recognise on that label, something that you can't actually describe, don't know what it's there for, or can't even pronounce—chances are it's not good for you.

The combination of ingredients in many energy drinks is actually rather frightening. Back when I was a young junior doctor, I remember seeing a patient in the emergency department experiencing acute psychosis. His friends told us he had consumed ten

---

8    Jari A. Laukkanen, "Sauna Use Associated with Reduced Risk of Cardiac, All-Cause Mortality," The JAMA Network, 2015, http://media.jamanetwork.com/news-item/sauna-use-associated-with-reduced-risk-of-cardiac-all-cause-mortality/.

energy drinks with vodka that night. He was hearing voices in his head instructing him that he should kill everyone around him and then kill himself. Not surprisingly, his friends became anxious and brought him to the hospital. After treating him with oxygen, intravenous fluids, cautious sedation, and overnight observations, he was back to normal with little recollection of the previous night's events. Obviously, that sort of madness isn't good for you.

If you feel you need an energy drink, ask yourself why. Why are you so low on energy that you'll guzzle down something that's potentially dangerous, that doesn't even really taste good, but which may give you a brief, drug-induced boost? Are the risks really worth it?

## CONSERVING ENERGY

This ties in with the Principle of Conservation of Energy, which states that "energy is neither created nor destroyed; it is merely converted from one form to another." For example, a light bulb transforms electrical energy to light energy. Conversely, a solar panel transforms light energy into electrical energy.

In keeping with this principle, if you're low on energy, chances are that you're either (1) not getting enough energy from your diet or environment, or (2) allowing your energy to be drained by external circumstances.

Be aware of your energy levels, and be conscious about how you're expending your energy. Are you getting healthy levels of air, water, and nutrients? What (or who) is sapping your energy? How can you address this imbalance?

You can stop putting your energy into doing things that really aren't serving your purpose or needs or doing anything positive for you. Think about where your energy is coming from and where it's going.

Find more ways to gain more energy from your diet and lifestyle. Natural foods will provide energy you can use straightaway.

Don't turn to caffeine and artificial stimulants when you are low on energy. Alternatively, I recommend taking deep diaphragmatic breaths and drinking a glass of water or freshly made juice. These actions work just like an energy shot. You'll feel much more awake. This provides steadier, long-lasting energy with no side effects or withdrawal a few hours later. It also helps you avoid the stomach acidity and reflux that caffeine can sometimes cause.

## ALCOHOL

Alcohol is a huge energy-drainer. If you have a hangover from drinking too much, you're basically suffering from a combination of dehydration and the toxic after-effects of alcohol. What's the most important thing you need to do to recover? Obviously drink water—lots of it. You need to replace the water lost from the diuretic effects of alcohol. Start drinking water immediately, slowly but steadily. After that, get some rest and put good nutrients back into your body.

Studies that support the health value of alcohol, especially red wine, are inconsistent at best. The general view seems to be that a daily glass of red wine probably won't hurt and could help your heart. I think it comes down not to medical advice but personal choice and the ability to limit your consumption to just that one glass each day. I like to keep things simple and based on common sense. Common sense says to me that more than one glass of wine a day isn't a sustainable long-term approach to balancing your health. Common sense also says that most forms of alcohol, including beer and distilled spirits, have a lot of stuff in them that is bad for your constitution.

## QUIT SMOKING

One of the most satisfying things I can do as a physician is to help a patient stop smoking. Your physical health depends upon what you put into your body. Putting the chemicals and carbon monoxide from cigarette smoke into your body and depriving your body of oxygen when you smoke is harmful. It does a lot of damage and has no sustained benefits.

### DOCTOR-FACILITATED SMOKING CESSATION

Doctors today tend to offer two options when prescribing methods to help patients stop smoking. Some prescribe nicotine-replacement therapy. Others prefer prescribing medications such as Varenicline and Bupropion. Both approaches have been found to have a degree of success. In my experience, nicotine replacement and drugs have mixed benefits. Some people find they're incredible and they work. Some have a relapse. Some find they don't work at all. Some people find the side effects too intolerable. There are other much safer therapeutic approaches, such as cognitive-behavioural therapy (CBT) or hypnosis. Alternatively, I highly recommend exploring the writings of Allen Carr or Bear Gebhardt, who have both written excellent books on smoking cessation.

### THE POWER OF SELF-MOTIVATION

There isn't anything quite as successful as a motivated individual who has a clear reason for quitting smoking and is absolutely committed to doing it. From that perspective, many different drug-free approaches can help. Many of these programs simply look at the source: Why do you smoke? Why do you want to stop? Quitting is easier when you understand why you're addicted and why you want to curb or abolish that addiction. Self-motivation and making the decision to stop also helps people avoid the expense and side effects of smoking-cessation drugs and nicotine replacement.

## TIMEFRAME

Everyone has a different timeframe for efforts to quit smoking. I have one patient who needed only a single hypnotherapy session to quit smoking for good. There are others who have tried many different types of smoking-cessation activities and weren't successful. Yet they haven't given up trying. The approaches to smoking cessation that work best vary with each person.

## MINDFULNESS AND MEDITATION

Regular practises of mindfulness, meditation, and clearing your emotional stress can reduce the desire and need for smoking. Mindfulness practises can give you a lot of insight into why you smoke and are discussed further in chapter 4. Supporting that with your compelling reasons for quitting and making a committed decision to throw out those cigarettes can yield great results.

Write down as many reasons as you can for stopping. Go beyond simple health reasons, such as avoiding lung disease, to deeper reasons, such as wanting to set a good example for your kids. Really explore why you genuinely, truly want to stop. That list can be hugely compelling.

My good friend Dillon recommends an approach he describes as the "100 Reasons Why." Write down one hundred reasons why you want to achieve your health goal (i.e., quitting smoking). This approach really gets you thinking and exploring your own perspectives. Take a moment to deeply contemplate, absorb and internalise each and every reason, one at a time. Eventually, amongst your one hundred reasons, you should find one or two (maybe more) that are truly compelling. This makes the process considerably easier. If you still can't find a compelling reason, write down one hundred more. Keep going until you find them. If your contemplation is deep enough, you'll get there.

Different people have different reasons for wanting to stop smoking. Some do it for their kids or their family. Others do it because they're sick of the colour of their fingernails or their stained teeth. Some do it because they want more energy or they want to sleep better or they want better skin. Complexion is actually one of the first things to improve when people stop smoking. It looks more radiant and fresher.

## TRIGGERS

In order to quit smoking, you must recognise what your smoking triggers are. Triggers can be emotions you attach to the cigarette. It doesn't become just about a cigarette. Leaving work to go outside and smoke becomes a private moment. The cigarette break becomes a little escape from the tumultuous day. You may go outside and smoke with your coworkers, in a secluded courtyard, or take a drive in your car. You may associate these breaks with socialization or precious moments of peace and quiet where you aren't bothered by the concerns or dramas of other people.

While someone is smoking, they're taking deep breaths in and trying to relax their mind, trying to be mindful, trying to connect with themselves. I emphasise the word "trying." Many people aren't all that successful at relaxing by smoking.

## SUBSTITUTING TRIGGERS

You can take that five minutes to do whatever you want to, but you don't have to pollute your lungs while you're doing it. Smoking during your personal time off is a conscious choice.

Whatever peace of mind and relaxation you achieve, or whatever activity you do while smoking a cigarette, you can also feel or do without a cigarette. You can remind yourself you need a little break and spend five minutes simply taking deep breaths and letting your thoughts settle. Doing so is a more effective method of relaxation and focus and is much healthier.

## TO MEDICATE OR NOT TO MEDICATE

I'm a great advocate of addressing lifestyle factors that contribute to disease. At the same time, as a doctor, I am an advocate of taking necessary medication when clinically appropriate. If your doctor has prescribed something for you, it's almost certainly for a very good reason, but make sure you fully understand what those reasons are. Involve your doctor in your positive lifestyle decisions, just as your doctor must involve you in any decisions to start medication. It's possible that by working together, you can reduce the amount of medication you may need.

For example, multiple sources indicate that 90 per cent of people with hypertension are diagnosed with "essential hypertension" or "primary hypertension," meaning no secondary cause can be found for it. You just have it, probably as a result of interplay between your genes and environment. In such cases, there's a lot you can do to lower your blood pressure without taking medicine. Your doctor may recommend lifestyle changes: improve your diet, eat fewer salty foods, stop smoking, lose weight, exercise more, and avoid stress. If you really do all those things, your blood pressure will likely decrease over a period of weeks or months. Unfortunately, a lot of people can't really manage to maintain those kinds of changes. Some would prefer to just take a daily pill (or two or three or even more) to bring their blood pressure down. Whilst doctors often do everything possible to support positive lifestyle decisions, the final choice rests with the patient. A doctor may prescribe the drugs as long as the patient is truly aware of benefits and the risks of taking drugs every day for the rest of his or her life.

Conversely, it is unfortunate that some doctors may suggest medication when all a patient requires is lifestyle changes. Be sure to ask your doctor if there are lifestyle changes you may try first, in lieu of medication, to improve your health conditions.

Some of the risks of medication aren't fully understood yet, because some of the newer drugs haven't been around long enough for us to really understand what they do. There's also a significant expense involved in taking at least one drug every day for many years. Many people need two or three drugs to control their blood pressure. I have known some patients who take up to five, six, and even seven drugs daily, and even then they are struggling.

Lifestyle changes don't need to be hard to make and sustain. It's easy to lose sight of why we want to make them. This is why I encourage the "100 Reasons Why" exercise. As long as you keep your reasons for wanting the changes in the forefront of your mind, then you'll have a much better chance of actively working towards your goals and ultimately reaching them.

## WEIGHT LOSS

One of the common areas people want to address when discussing health is their physical appearance and desire to lose weight. Some weight gain may be genetic. However, what you eat and how much exercise you get will certainly contribute to your weight. You can't change your genes, but everyone can improve their diet and exercise regime.

Of course, realistically, no one has the perfect diet or the perfect exercise program. So the goal here is not to worry about perfection but to focus on improvement. Look at what you eat and how much exercise you take. If you're still putting on weight, chances are you're either doing too much of the first or not enough of the second. When people take a natural approach to changing food habits and truly address the question of exercise, they'll generally find they lose weight.

I often hear patients say they're overweight because of their genes. They tell me, "I can't help it. You can't fight your genes." It's not really a matter of fighting your genes. It's about doing what you can to support your body. The genes will do what the genes will do, but you can give yourself a fighting chance at losing weight and preventing or postponing related illness.

Our social well-being can also influence how successful we are in improving our health. If we surround ourselves with people who are overweight, their behaviours will influence us. It's very hard for a husband to lose weight if his wife is clearly not interested in eating healthy herself, and the same is true when the roles are reversed. Couples who make a joint effort to lose weight and truly commit to the effort are much more likely to reach their goal weights. We will explore social well-being later in chapter 6.

CHAPTER 3

_____

# ACTIVITY AND REST

The human body is designed to be active. We're not designed to be sedentary and stuck in an office or by a computer all day and all night, or even worse, glued to a TV set or a smartphone. The actual physiology of the human body is designed for us to move. Throughout most of human history, we were very active—we had to be to survive. But in the present, we now have less and less reasons to move. Everything is extremely convenient. For example, you can now buy a pizza on your mobile-phone app, and it will be delivered to your door within thirty minutes. You can also look on your phone to find out what stage of preparation your pizza is in while you're waiting. You don't need to speak to anyone or move from your couch.

It's no longer viewed as necessary for many of us to partake in regular physical activity—it is no longer a normal and integral part of many people's lives. Accordingly, your body, because it is not moving, stagnates. Your blood and lymph systems don't circulate so well, so lymph collects and isn't properly eliminated. Bowel motions can become less frequent. Your lungs aren't working to their full capacity because they don't need to. You're not necessarily getting enough oxygen. And because your muscles aren't moving, the blood flow to them is reduced. If your muscles don't need to work so hard, they actually start to atrophy—they decrease in size and waste away.

In the Western world, our average daily calorie consumption is far above what human beings actually require on a day-to-day basis, particularly those who have a sedentary lifestyle. Those extra calories can get converted to fat, making obesity a prevalent health problem.

Nobody can really define what the right amount of nourishment or exercise is. In my opinion, this is a real problem. In general, we can probably say that if someone is persistently overweight, they're likely getting too much nourishment and not enough of exercise. Addressing that imbalance will start to work in their favour and help them achieve their health and weight goals.

Increasing your activity level simply makes you feel better. This has been proven in many published scientific studies. You may lose weight, improve your circulation, get rid of waste better, and feel stronger. Activity is also a very good way to work through emotional disturbances or imbalances. Many studies show us that depression and anxiety can both be improved by regular exercise.

## MODERATE EXERCISE

*"Those who think they have no time for exercise will sooner or later have to find time for illness."*

### —Edward Stanley

Few of us are really, truly participating in the level of activity we need. My advice here is short and simple: undertake some form of physical activity every single day for thirty minutes.

Each of us can find thirty minutes in a day to do something that gets us moving. You don't need to go to the gym or even leave the house. You can easily ride an exercise bike or do a simple workout with kettle bells or dumbells. Use a rebounder, or even do simple chair exercises while you watch TV. Rebounders, or mini trampolines, have been shown to improve muscle tone, blood and lymph circulation, bone density, and coordination. They give you a great aerobic exercise that works almost every muscle in the body. In my experience, rebounding can burn a hundred calories in less than ten minutes, and it doesn't even feel like exercise. I would highly recommend purchasing one and using it every day.

It's vital to create time for exercise every single day, if possible. Unfortunately, with our busy schedules that are often so geared towards meeting other people's needs, we so easily neglect our own. To correct that imbalance, you may need to put yourself first a bit more. Think of it this way: To meet all those needs, you need to meet your own first. Remind yourself, *I need to be strong, I need to be fit, I need to be healthy—so I need to undertake some amount of activity every day.*

Keep your activity to a level that is comfortable and enjoyable for you. I recommend against trying to do too much too soon. If you decide that running is the activity that you'd like to try, there's no need to run a marathon, or even half a mile, on your first day. You'll probably feel really stiff the next day, and you're a lot less likely to stick with any activity that's painful. If you want to enjoy your activity, approach it with reasonable expectations. If you're out of condition, set a simple, small, achievable goal. You might need to start just by walking once around the block.

You have three exercise goals: to get slightly out of breath, increase your heart rate, and work up a little sweat. If you're reaching those three areas, then that's a good amount of aerobic exercise and activity. Just walking is sometimes enough to reach the three goals.

Your exercise pace should be substantial enough that you can talk but not sing.

Research shows that while thirty minutes of exercise is crucial, it doesn't have to be thirty minutes in a row. You might do fifteen minutes at lunch time by taking a walk and another fifteen at home with your rebounder or weights or taking another walk. If you can't manage the second fifteen minutes that day, it's not the end of the world or a reason to give up on increasing your activity. Make it up the next day if you want. It's more important to just get back on the thirty-minutes-a-day track.

## PRIVATE SPACE

I find that creating some activity time for myself is a way to not only practise mindfulness but is also a gift to myself. I'm taking care of myself and also giving myself that thirty minutes of carved out space. I don't answer the phone or check emails or talk with anyone during my workout. I tend to do it early in the morning while my family is still asleep, but when I do it at other times, I ask them not to interrupt. They mostly respect my wishes and understand how important that workout time is to me. Of course, stuff happens, especially if you have children. My goal isn't to have a perfect workout for thirty uninterrupted minutes a day, but it is to get in activity on a regular basis. Again, if you can manage this 80 per cent of the time or even 50 per cent of the time, you're doing fantastic. Don't worry about the days you miss.

You don't have to join a gym to be active. Going to the gym works well for some—they appreciate the equipment, enjoy the camaraderie, and like working with a trainer. Others don't want to spend the money, don't live or work somewhere convenient to a gym, prefer a private workout, or just don't want the commitment. I've joined several different gyms over the years. It's interesting to see certain people there all the time, looking exactly the same month after month, year after year. They don't actually seem to have changed their physical appearance, lost weight, or to have built muscle. That tells me that either they're not exercising correctly or that a gym membership will not always get what you want in terms of greater health.

## ONE FOOT IN FRONT OF THE OTHER

A study presented in 2015 at the European Society of Cardiology (ESC) Congress showed that twenty-five minutes of brisk walking a day could add up to seven years to your life and halve the risk of dying from a heart attack.[9] If there was a pill that could do that with no side effects, all my patients would be asking for it, and I'd be happy to prescribe it. Instead, I prescribe walking. It's much better than a pill because it's free and has no side effects. You don't need any special training or any equipment. You can walk anywhere that's safe for you, at any time that's good for you. In my experience, there's no reason why anyone can't find twenty-five minutes in their daily schedule for a walk if they're able-bodied.

There are many theories about why a daily walk helps your health. The theories touch upon stress hormones, biomechanics, increased oxygen intake, and other physiological changes. Personally I'm not too interested in the theories. I'm more interested in the fact that it works. It works, so let's start doing it. Let's recognise the connection between walking and feeling better and really use it for our benefit.

---

9    Paul Peachey, "A daily walk 'can add several years to your life,'" August 30, 2015, www.independent.co.uk/life-style/health-and-families/health-news/a-daily-walk-can-add-seven-years-to-your-life-10478821.html.

Some people enjoy walking with a group. Knowing that the group is waiting for you can make you join them even when you're not really feeling much like walking. If you're with a good peer group consisting of people who all have good intentions to improve their health, then walking with that group can really increase your pleasure and help you to forge positive social connections. Other people like to walk with just one other person or with family members. Some prefer to walk alone to get some personal time. If you think a group would help you walk more regularly, then by all means try it. If you find you don't enjoy group walking and prefer to walk alone, walk alone.

I believe time isn't something we have, but rather, it's something we create. We can create time for anything if we decide it's important enough. If you decide your health and well-being are important enough, finding thirty minutes to walk or exercise should not a problem.

A few of my patients really struggle with mobility. They can't walk much or at all, but I encourage them to find other enjoyable activities. If you can't walk or do a gym workout—let's say you have bad knee arthritis, for instance—you can, in many cases, still be active. Keep your focus on what you *can* do and the benefits of activity—not on what limits you. One of my most inspirational patients is confined to a wheelchair, but he helps coach the GB Olympic wheelchair basketball team. He's always very joyous and self-sufficient, and he's very, very fit. Whenever I try to help him by opening a door, he always stops me, "No, no. I've got it."

I actually prefer to see my patients walk or swim instead of run. Regular prolonged running can be quite hazardous to the hips and knees because of the impact it has on those joints. Swimming and water aerobics are great if you can't put a lot of weight on your legs.

Swimming solves that problem because it's not a high-impact activity. It's very relaxed and fluid; it's good for the joints. Swimming is a great activity for anyone. It exercises every muscle in your body and gets them all moving. I know from my patients (and also my mother) that it's never too late to learn how to swim.

## GYM PRESCRIPTIONS

As a physician, I'm able to prescribe exercise to my patients. We can prescribe a gym membership for twelve weeks to our patients. The gyms love it because in theory, after someone has been coming in for free for twelve weeks, they will be fitter and will, one hopes, enjoy the workouts. They then stay on and join the gym as a member. Disappointingly, few people ask for the gym prescription. Of those who do, even fewer actually follow through. It's very rare that I prescribe a gym membership and see the patient go through the full twelve-week program. You don't need a prescription gym membership to be healthier.

I often hear from my patients that exercise is boring. Well, it can be, unless you find a way to make it enjoyable. Put on some good music or listen to an audiobook or watch TV. Find an exercise partner. Anything at all that you can do to keep yourself suitably entertained while you're exercising is absolutely vital because that will help you stick with a routine.

## SETTING GOALS

I learned a lot about exercise when I asked my wife to marry me in February 2006, and we set the date for September. I thought, *I've really got to get myself into shape now. I don't want to be an overweight groom.*

I got into the best shape of my life because I had good reason. I wanted to look good on the most important day of my life. I wanted to make sure I looked like someone who deserved to marry such a beautiful woman. I was hitting the gym every single day. I adopted my old friend's mantra: "My day is not complete until I have exercised." I got myself into incredible shape, simply because I had established a clear reason *why* I needed to.

The most amazing insight I found at the gym was that my energy levels spiked. Prior to becoming a regular exerciser, I would need to have a little snooze in the late afternoon or early evening every day just to replenish my energy. Napping stopped after I became a regular exerciser. I started drinking more water during that time and taking daily essential fatty acid supplements. I quickly noticed improvements in my skin and hair, and for the first time I did not get any hay fever symptoms that summer.

Each little thing you do for your health might seem small, but when you put them together consistently over time, they compound. Darren Hardy talks about this in his great book *The Compound Effect*. Small positive changes compounded can have a huge impact on your overall physical health, appearance, and on your emotions over time. When you look good and are strong, you feel confident—and when you feel confident, you can stick with your diet and exercise.

Setting achievable and realistic goals is most important, but you must also measure your progress. It's easy to track your activity level and compare it to how you feel and how you look. When you start to see the results, you'll want to continue to measure and manage.

Most people who are overweight don't want to lose weight. They want to lose fat. You don't want to lose weight from vital organic tissues like your liver or your bones or your muscles. You specifically want to lose fat, so fat is what you should measure. You can buy an inexpensive, handheld body fat monitor you can easily use at home or a scale that gives your weight and body composition. You want to know not just your weight but also what your body fat percentage is. How lean do you ideally want to be?

Using your actual weight and your body fat percentage, you can calculate how much fat you are carrying. For example, if you weigh 100kg and your body fat percentage is 25%, you are carrying 25kg of body fat. If fat loss is your goal, I would recommend you monitor and manage this latter figure, rather than your overall weight. I track my weight and body fat percentage using a spreadsheet that works out the weight of my body fat compared to the rest of my weight. Using the spreadsheet, I can also figure out what my lean body mass is, meaning how much I weigh if I take away the fat. I monitor that on a regular basis. Seeing the numbers is a good motivator.

In general, if you stick to a sensible, healthy diet, are active for thirty minutes a day, and drink plenty of water, you will gradually see the percentage of your body fat drop. You will be able to see how much of the weight loss is fat. Once you see those numbers start to fall, it's incredibly encouraging. This can help to motivate you to continue working towards your weight-loss goals.

If you don't see the numbers drop, don't get discouraged. You've got the plan, and it will work. Try to pinpoint where the imbalance is. Are you truly eating a good diet, spending thirty minutes a day being active, and drinking lots of water? The imbalance is probably somewhere in there.

Using a spreadsheet is a great way to monitor your progress. I recommend checking the spreadsheet at least once a week, preferably on the same day every week. If you want to be more extreme, you can monitor yourself every day.

Weigh yourself first thing in the morning, undressed, after you've used the bathroom. Check your weight and body fat percentage, and enter them into the spreadsheet. If you do this consistently every day or every week on the same day, you'll start to see patterns and get a much better sense of whether or not the numbers are corresponding with your goals. If they're not, then review your plan and make sure that you're truly sticking to your plan.

I believe objective measurements are important for helping you gauge how the steps you take lead to improvement. You can easily track your blood pressure, your heart rate, and your weight and body fat percentage at home with appropriate monitors. Some of my patients use activity tracker devices and apps such as Fitbit, and there is some scientific evidence to support their use. Whether these are truly accurate may be open to debate, but they're probably close enough to make them worthwhile.[10] Do you need to quantify how much exercise you get? The amount of activity that's right is personal. It's more important to measure the results than to measure the process.

## WEIGHT LOSS

A healthy weight loss rate is one to two pounds, or about a kilo, per week. Dramatic weight loss of more than four pounds a week suggests you're probably eating an unhealthy diet without enough calories and nutrition. In addition to losing fat, you may be losing muscle or tissue from vital organs, so your lean body weight goes down. That's unhealthy.

---

10    Liam G. Glynn, Patrick S. Hayes, Monica Casey, Fergus Glynn, Alberto Alvarez-Iglesias, John Newell, Gearóid ÓLaighin, David Heaney, Martin O'Donnell, Andrew W. Murphy, "Effectiveness of a smartphone application to promote physical activity in primary care: the SMART MOVE randomized controlled trial," *British Journal of General Practice*, 2014, doi: 10.3399/bjgp14X680461.

Sometimes your weight loss will just stall. You hit a plateau. This can be discouraging, but it's also normal. Your body is essentially saying, "Hold on, I need a little break here." Take a day off from the plan. Have a break day where you just take it easy. Don't deviate dramatically from the plan, and don't overindulge, but maybe eat something that's a treat. Hit the plan again the next day.

Your weight might go up a little bit after a break day, but that's okay. Getting off the plateau will get your weight loss moving again. Weight will start to come off at the same rate it did before. To help get off a plateau and keep losing weight, keep drinking plenty of water. On average, this requires two to three litres a day.

## WHAT DOES HEALTH LOOK LIKE?

At the start of chapter 1, we discussed the definition of health, and I invited you to consider what being truly healthy would look like to you and to write down five personal reasons why you want better health. If you skipped this part, please revisit this, as your reasons why can be the most essential component to achieving the health you desire.

For example, one of my dear friends decided that making some positive lifestyle changes would help her confidence and self-esteem. She started off with a healthy detox that included organic foods, fresh juices, water, meditation, yoga, gentle activity, deep-breathing exercises, and colonic irrigation. Basically, she cleared her mind and body of some of the physical and emotional waste she was carrying—that's all a detox is. Most importantly, she then maintained the healthy habits she had learned. Just letting go of so much of the waste her body was carrying every day and putting in the good nutrients that give our cells what they need to survive really transformed everything for her. She got her energy back, to the point where she needed a lot less sleep. Not only did she look and feel better, but she told me her personal income also went up four-fold that year. She believes this was all because of the lifestyle changes. Her friends were a little sceptical, especially about the cleanse and colon part. However, when she told them about her increased income, it certainly got their attention.

Does doing a detox make you rich? Not necessarily, but making positive lifestyle changes that work for you to get your energy and self-confidence back will certainly make you richer in health. It may well give you more clarity about your life's direction, as it certainly did for my friend. Knowing *why* you want to get to your goal is the most important part of deciding to get healthier. Once you deeply understand and take ownership of your personal *why*, the ways to achieve your goal will follow.

## GETTING THE SLEEP YOU NEED

I'm a great believer in getting enough sleep. I'm not a big fan of alarm clocks going off, dragging yourself out of bed to go to work, and then needing three cups of coffee just to function. If that's you, then what you need isn't more coffee but more sleep. More balance.

One of the most common complaints I hear from patients is, "I'm tired all the time." On occasion, there may be medical causes for this, but the vast majority of the time the solution is very simple: sleep more, and then review your energy intake and expenditure. Are you getting enough energy from your diet, lifestyle, and environment? Are you putting too much energy into some of your daily tasks? Many of us don't get the sleep that we deserve and need every single night. Accordingly, as I discussed earlier, many of us are in a sleep deficit—we owe our bodies for the sleep we're not getting. If you're sleep-deprived, you can try to make up for it on the weekends, but it's not really all that easy, especially if you have small children.

Good-quality sleep, where you fall asleep quickly and stay asleep for at least several hours and fall asleep again quickly if you wake in the night, is absolutely vital. Your body and your brain need that restful time to repair and recover. Good-quality sleep often only occurs if you've been sufficiently physically active during the day and if you take time to deactivate your brain before you go to sleep at night. Sleep isn't just about physical rest. It's also about mental rest.

## INSOMNIA

Everybody's going to have the occasional night where, for whatever reason, whether it is jet lag or family worries, they can't sleep. They might feel a little groggy the next day, but the next night, they will fall asleep quickly or go to bed a bit earlier because they are so tired.

Such is not the case for sufferers of insomnia, which is generally defined as habitual poor sleep more often than not over the course of several weeks, or as poor sleep at least three times a week for at least three months. Among my patients, the vast majority of the time insomnia is a symptom of something else. It's a symptom of the body being out of balance, often because of mental or emotional stress, poor diet, or lack of exercise. Restoring that balance will eliminate the insomnia.

## SLEEPING PILLS

Some years ago, doctors used to liberally prescribe sleeping tablets for insomnia. Sleeping drugs will almost inevitably make you feel somewhat drowsy the next day. Some manufacturers claim this doesn't happen, but these drugs affect your brain. Some parts of your brain will be sluggish the next day. That's not a state that you want to be in if you want to be at your best the following day. It used to be relatively easy to get your doctor to prescribe sleeping drugs, but today doctors prescribe such tablets rarely, simply because of the side effects. You can develop a tolerance for sleeping drugs and need ever-increasing doses and suffer ever-accumulating side effects. You can even become addicted. Sleeping pills that are popular when they first come out end up being taken off the market or become a lot less popular once the side effects become noticeable.

Rather than sleeping drugs, today we work with our patients on what we call sleep hygiene (which has nothing to do with cleanliness). Sleep hygiene refers to your sleep habits and your approach to sleep, which basically revert to your cycle of activity and rest. General recommendations include avoiding daytime naps, exercising early in the day, avoiding consuming stimulants like caffeine, avoiding physical or mental exertion before sleep, limiting worrying, avoiding large meals before sleep, and also actually getting out of bed if sleep does not naturally come. Of all of these, I feel the most effective is to focus on mental rest—allowing your thoughts to settle while taking gentle breaths and moving away from worrying thoughts.

## RE-ANGLING THE STORY

I once had a young patient who came to see me with her brother. At the end of her consultation, the brother said to me, "Quick question, Doc, I can't sleep at night. What do I do?"

I said, "What's keeping you awake?"

He replied, "I've got all these thoughts and things going on in my head. I'm just worrying all the time." He described troublesome thoughts coming to mind and how a trigger of sorts was pulled, and those thoughts would just keep flowing through his mind and turn into even more worrying thoughts.

I simply reminded him that he was the only person in control of his thoughts: he could decide what he thought about and when he thought about those things. I suggested he come up with a list of more positive, relaxing thoughts to start thinking about when approaching the time for sleep.

By thinking through the problem with the patient and asking him why he allowed these thoughts to come when it was time for his mind to rest, he decided to work on reining in those sleep-disrupting thoughts. He was able to take corrective action for his insomnia, without drugs. He went off and implemented a solution. He took full ownership of the problem, and it worked.

## DIFFICULT NIGHTS

When you're in bed at the end of the night, a train of thought can sometimes start to roll in. One thought leads to another thought, which leads to yet another thought. Particularly worrying or distressing images you're creating can keep you awake. Then you look at the clock and see it's two in the morning. You think, *I've got to be up in four hours.* That thought creates even more stress and makes you even more sleepless.

### BREAKING INTERRUPTED SLEEP PATTERNS

To get better sleep, it's important to break that bedtime pattern. The first step is just to recognise that there is a pattern. Step two is to break it by realizing that there's only one person in the world who controls what you think about, and that's you. You can *choose* what you are going to think about and deliberately only filter in calm, restful, relaxing thoughts for the night.

An exercise I often recommend for helping you fall asleep is focusing on gratitude. The benefits of practising gratitude are increasingly being studied and have already been well documented in numerous books by renowned professor of psychology, Dr

Robert Emmons. As you lie in bed before sleep, think about things you're grateful for, that you perhaps take for granted every day but would struggle without. That can put you into a very relaxed state that lets your mind settle. Focus on calming thoughts and taking gentle breaths.

## 4–7–8 BREATHING

Another good method for getting to sleep quickly is called the 4–7–8 breathing technique. The origins of this technique are thought to be yogic, and it was popularised by Dr Andrew Weil, a leader in integrative medicine. 4–7–8 breathing can put you to sleep in sixty seconds or a few minutes at most. If you have trouble falling asleep, it's certainly worth trying. It works well for some of my patients— and it works well for me.

Once you're comfortably in bed and have allowed your thoughts to settle, exhale completely through your mouth. Then close your mouth and inhale through your nose for a count of four. Hold your breath for a count of seven. Exhale completely through your mouth for a count of eight. Repeat the cycle again as needed.

Frankly, I don't know how this works. It may work because it keeps your mind focused on your breathing and nothing else. You're mindful. The mind is quiet and settled. You're also getting a good amount of oxygen when you breathe in, and you're eliminating a good amount of waste when you breathe out.

I'd much rather recommend the 4–7–8 breathing method for a couple of weeks than just hand over a prescription for a sleeping medication. I'd also advise against nonprescription drugs such as antihistamines. No drug, prescription or otherwise, is without side effects.

## HOW MUCH SLEEP DO YOU NEED?

How much sleep is enough? The number of hours of sleep needed varies according to the individual. If you feel refreshed and ready for the day in the morning, then you probably slept long enough. Six to eight hours is the average number of hours most people need to feel rested.

To get a more accurate idea of how much sleep you need personally, try going to bed a little earlier in the evening and do whatever works for you to help you fall asleep quickly. Note when you naturally wake up the next morning. Did you wake up before your alarm? Note how you feel. Do you feel refreshed? Are you able to get through your day well, without feeling tired? Keep track of your sleep until you find the sleep duration that seems to be right for you. That number may change over time.

It is important to know your basic sleep needs/requirements and be sure you meet them. Countless studies have shown that sleep deprivation can harm or adversely affect performance the next day and has also been linked with diabetes and obesity. Drowsy driving is a very serious hazard, just as serious as driving drunk. If you're constantly having to drag yourself out of bed every day, or if you hit snooze on your alarm clock more than twice, perhaps it's time to give your body what it needs—more sleep.

Once you have achieved balance nutritionally, begun an exercise regime, and rebalanced your sleep debt, you will find that your sleep requirement actually reduces. You might get to the point where you have a productive day following six hours or less of sleep per night.

## FINDING A SUSTAINABLE PATTERN

When I was a young doctor in training, there were times when I would get home and literally fall into a heap in my bed. It would feel like I had barely been asleep for about five or ten minutes. Then my alarm clock would go off and I would realize it was the next day. I'd think, *Is that all the sleep I get?* It was.

I'd be back at work thirty minutes later thinking, *This is not sustainable.* In the long run, it wasn't, but that was the choice I had made because I wanted to be in medicine. Even after I became a partner in my practice and had greater control over my hours, I still sometimes worked late in the evenings, and I'd always be gone in the morning before everyone else was awake. Eventually, I found ways to work more efficiently and make sure that my work was completed on time so I could leave on time and be with my family. But after a while I asked myself: *Do I need to work this many hours? How can I step back a little? What can I do so I can spend more time with my family without reducing my income?*

I didn't want to spend my whole life working as a doctor up to seven days per week, constantly feeling tired. I made some lifestyle changes. It wasn't easy, but it was absolutely worth it.

The important thing here is to know what you want. Do you want to have more time with your family? Do you want to make more money? Do you want to travel the world? Or all three?

An interesting meta-analysis published in 2005 revealed that more people die from a sudden cardiac event on a Monday than any other day of the week.[11] Why do you think this may be?

It's important to make choices that will fulfil you and make you happy. If you're doing something professionally that is not enjoyable or that is draining your energy without offering any fulfilment, then consider a different approach. From a health perspective, it's important to have passion for what you're doing professionally. If

11    D.R. Witte, D.E. Grobbee, M.L. Bots, and A.W. Hoes, "A meta-analysis of excess cardiac mortality on Monday," *European Journal of Epidemiology* 20 (2005): 401–406, doi: 10.1007/s10654-004-8783-6.

you're not really truly aligned with what your company or organisation represents and how you're serving your community, then you may start to feel detached from it. You may start to see your job *only* as a means to make money to pay your bills and support your family. Wouldn't it be better to have a job that is truly aligned with what you are passionate about as a person, that you feel is serving and helping people—but that also pays your bills and provides downtime to spend with your family? I know that's easier said than done. I'm not suggesting it's easy, but once you find or create this kind of role, you may find it was really worth it.

# CHAPTER 4

# FINDING EMOTIONAL BALANCE

*"If you realised how powerful your thoughts are, you would never think a negative thought again."*

## —Peace Pilgrim (Mildred Lisette Norman)

Our emotions—our feelings of joy, love, gratitude, anger, sorrow, fear—arise from the thoughts we have day to day and how we process them. In his excellent book *Quantum Healing*, Dr. Deepak Chopra describes that the average human being is estimated to have around sixty thousand thoughts per day, but that 95 per cent of those thoughts are ones we had the previous day.[12] That's really surprising. How many of those thoughts are really serving us, and how many are actually harming us? How many of those thoughts are causing undue distress?

*"You become what you think about all day long."*

## —Ralph Waldo Emerson

---

12  Deepak Chopra, *Quantum Healing* (New York: Bantam, 1990).

Your thoughts can be extremely powerful because they can actually have a physiological effect on your body. Focusing your thoughts on a positive level and creating positive emotions can lead your body to secrete more endorphins, serotonin, and dopamine, amongst other hormones and neurotransmitters. Positive thoughts help to create calmness, uplift you, and increase your energy levels throughout the day. This has been studied in the field of psychoneuroimmunology, which explores the interactions between the nervous and immune systems and the relationship between behaviour and health.

If you think sufficiently or intensely enough about something positive—how much you love your child, for instance—you can actually feel it within your body. That's because your thought is triggering off certain hormones, neurotransmitters, and biochemical reactions within your body chemistry that cause you to feel that way.

Conversely, negative thoughts also cause a physiological reaction. If you truly focus your thoughts on someone who's wronged you or harmed you or betrayed you in the past, and you really think about those events at a very, very, deep level, then you can also start to feel that agitation in your body as a result. This happens because you're firing off various hormones and neurotransmitters, such as noradrenaline, cortisol, and inflammatory mediators.

Naturally, it is in our body's best interest to refocus on positive thoughts. Positive thoughts may include gratitude, past achievements, and exciting future plans. Gratitude is an incredibly powerful emotion; when you feel grateful for something, that feeling can stir up many chemical changes within your system. Positive emotions such as gratitude increase serotonin and dopamine levels in the brain, which also make you feel calmer. Positive emotions also help bring down blood pressure, relax your muscles, and relieve anxiety and depression. Studies show that thinking positively and focussing on gratitude can also help support cardiac health in people with heart disease.[13]

## THE VALUE OF MEDITATION

*"You should sit in meditation for twenty minutes a day—unless you're too busy. Then you should sit for an hour."*

### —Zen proverb

Many patients come to me for help because they feel overwhelmed by racing thoughts. It's certainly distressing when your brain feels like it's in a sandstorm and so many thoughts are occupying your mind, all vying for your attention. Mindfulness and meditative practises can help the sandstorm to pass—your thoughts settle down, and you start to feel in control again.

I would recommend meditation for everyone. It's actually an incredibly simple activity. I believe anyone can learn the basics in five minutes. I've never met anyone who practises meditation regularly and claims it doesn't help.

Meditation is simply time spent in quiet contemplation. Beyond that, there are no rules or requirements. Meditation turns out to be easy, something that anyone can do pretty much anywhere. With some practise, you can even meditate on a noisy bus ride.

Start simple, start easy. A regular meditation practise only requires you to find a quiet place where you won't be disturbed for twenty minutes or so. Turn off your phone. Tell everyone around

13   Paul J. Mills, Deepak Chopra, Laura Redwine, Kathleen Wilson, Meredith A. Pung, Kelly Chin, Barry H. Greenberg, Ottar Lunde, Alan Maisel, Ajit Raisinghani, and Alex Wood, "The Role of Gratitude in Spiritual Well-Being in Asymptomatic Heart Failure Patients," *Spirituality in Clinical Practice* 2 (2015): 5–17, http://dx.doi.org/10.1037/scp0000050.

you to leave you alone, close the door if possible, and sit down in a comfortable place.

Close your eyes. Take some deep breaths in and out, and then just be present with whatever thoughts surface in your mind during the moment. Don't push any thoughts away. Don't force any new thoughts in. Just be present with whatever thoughts are there in the moment.

Set it up so that you're just meditating on your own, uninterrupted, for at least twenty minutes. Just be with whatever thoughts are present in the moment. Keep your eyes closed, and breathe deeply and comfortably. Keep your body still, and then let the mind become still. Allow yourself to just be with whatever thought arises in the moment. Let that thought do what it wants to do, allow it to settle, and just keep your mind as still as you can. Be aware of the thoughts that arise, simply as an observer. Don't express them or suppress them. Don't magnify them or push them away. Let thoughts arise; let them settle.

In this relaxed state of mind, you may find that you get good ideas and inspiration. The solution to a problem at work might just arise in your mind, without you having to consciously think about it. Great ideas can arise from the mental stillness.

Keeping your mind still like this for just twenty minutes or so can have an incredible calming effect on the body and the mind. Meditation helps clear and relax your mind. You remain awake and alert while you meditate, but your mind is focused inwardly. As you leave that meditative state, you will probably find yourself in a much calmer state. You have essentially helped clear some of the emotional stress that you may have been carrying.

Guided meditation helps some people get started on a regular meditation practise. Guided meditations walk you through a meditation session one step at a time. A lot of free guided meditations of varying lengths, often with soothing music, are found online and on YouTube. You can easily download sessions onto your phone or tablet. If you decide to get started this way, find a quiet place where you won't be interrupted and just listen with earphones. The recordings will help you through a pretty straightforward session. Most people who start with guided meditation can then easily move on to independent meditation without the support.

Many people like to repeat a mantra, a word or sound that aids concentration in meditation. Your mantra can be anything you want it to be so long as it supports your state. Examples may include repeating the word "calm" or "relax"—choose a mantra that resonates with you. But a mantra is also optional. If solely focusing on your breathing keeps you in that relaxed state, that's fine. I recommend aiming for a minimum of twenty uninterrupted minutes a day.

Meditating on a regular basis can improve conditions such as hypertension and chronic pain. It can also improve your brain function, creativity, intelligence, and your performance professionally and academically. There's even some evidence that regular meditation can increase longevity.[14]

## VISUALIZATION

Another approach to meditation is visualization. This is something a lot of athletes and performers use as a way to simultaneously relax and improve their skills. Find a quiet place and relax by focusing

---

14   Brook, Robert D. et al., "Beyond Medications and Diet: Alternative Approaches to Lowering Blood Pressure. A Scientific Statement from the American Heart Association", April 22, 2013; Duraimani S et al. (2015) "Effects of Lifestyle Modification on Telomerase Gene Expression in Hypertensive Patients: A Pilot Trial of Stress Reduction and Health Education Programs"; Kabat-Zinn et al "The clinical use of mindfulness meditation for the self-regulation of chronic pain" Behav Med (1985).

on your breathing. As you feel yourself relaxing, imagine yourself, in great detail, performing an activity you wish to do. In one study, the participants were basketball players who wanted to improve their three-point shots. One group was assigned to practise shooting from outside the circle for an hour every day for two weeks. The other group was assigned to spend an hour in silent meditation, visualising themselves shooting outside the circle, for an hour every day. At the end of fourteen days, the two groups had a shoot-off. The results were identical. One group actively practised three-point shots, while the other just visualised them, yet both landed their baskets equally well.[15]

Visualization is also helpful for more common activities. You might be worried about making a presentation at work, for example. Spending some time visualising yourself making that presentation every day for several days before the event can really help you feel calm and confident about doing it. Thoroughly imagine every step of the process, from stepping in front of the group, to delivering your speech, to thanking everyone and walking away. It will be almost exactly as if you were actually doing it, but you can stop and think about every step along the way. Of course, visualisation is not a substitute for good preparation beforehand, but it is clearly a powerful way to support the process.

You can also use visualisation to relieve stress by imagining yourself in a place or doing something that you find pleasant and relaxing. Again, begin as if you were starting to meditate. Then imagine your favourite place, in as much detail as you can. If it's the beach, focus on your surroundings. Feel the warmth of the sun, touch the sand, and hear the sound of the surf. The more you focus

---

15    L.V. Clark, "Effect of mental practice on the development of a certain motor skill," *Research Quarterly* 31 (1960): 560–569, doi: 10.2190/X9BA-KJ68-07AN-QMJ8.

on the enjoyable aspects of whatever place you choose, the more your worries and concerns fade away. When you leave your visualisation, you may find that you now feel more relaxed, have a better perspective on life, and are in a stronger position to address any problems.

## AFFIRMATIONS

Affirmations are another tool for focusing your mind and relieving stress. Many people use affirmations. Think of a very clear, direct, positive statement, in the present tense, of what you want to achieve. An example might be, "I am strong," or, "I am productive." Repeat your affirmation to yourself whenever you can. An affirmation can move you towards the mental and emotional state you require to achieve your goals.

If you're working on losing weight and building muscle, your affirmation might be something that supports your decision. You might say, "I am burning fat, and I am building muscle." Or just cut it down to something simple, "Burning fat, building muscle." While you're at the gym, repeating that phrase over and over again can motivate you to complete your workout and maybe even step it up. Try it. Compare your week-by-week results while repeating affirmations versus not repeating affirmations and see how different the results can be. You may see quite a significant improvement.

## LEARNING MORE ABOUT MEDITATION

If you want to learn more about the many ways you can meditate and find some basic instruction and ideas, visit the website *www.tm.org*, which is run by the Maharishi Foundation, a nonprofit educational organisation. The site has excellent information, including a lot about the health benefits of regular meditation. They offer inexpensive courses teaching their most effective way of meditation, which I would recommend. However, I believe there is no right or wrong way to meditate; just do it, and you'll get better at it. The more you understand about meditation, however, the sooner you can find effective ways to do it. You don't need a teacher to learn to meditate, but some people find that a brief class or session with an instructor helps to get started. To find a class or instructor, check with your local community, health clubs, and personal trainers. You may be surprised at how easy it is to find someone to guide you.

Meditation, visualisation, and affirmations are all great practises to help with emotional well-being and restoring balance. Because the mind is quiet while you meditate, your inner thoughts can start to materialise. Many people have told me they get some of their best ideas from being in a meditative state. I've also found that to be true.

## NEGATIVE EMOTIONS

*"I learned that illness wasn't random and wasn't genetic for the most part...In fact most illnesses can be traced to certain emotional patterns."*

**—Dr Gabor Maté, physician, author, speaker**

How much of our time do we spend focusing on negative emotions such as regret, anger, frustration, jealousy, betrayal, criticism, and self-criticism? Many of those emotions don't serve us well. They can actually create a chemical imbalance within our bodies, which can have an adverse effect on our health. Our emotional well-being will be much improved if we can address the negativity that we consciously or unconsciously embrace. A good starting point is just identifying and labelling your negative emotions. Make a list, look at it, and ask yourself how those feelings are serving you. The truth is, they're often not. Instead, they can have the opposite effect. These feelings can drain your physical and emotional energy.

Let go of them and replace them with more positive thoughts, focusing on gratitude, the abundance you already have, past achievements, things that you're looking forward to, things that you enjoy, things you're passionate about, people you love, and the people who love you. When you truly focus on positive thoughts, you energise yourself. This is a very powerful way to help restore your energy and well-being and eliminate stress.

Dr Emmet Fox wrote a very short but excellent book describing this area called *The Seven Day Mental Diet*, which is freely available on the Internet. I would recommend seeking out this book now and reading it before you go any further—it should only take ten minutes.

## POSTURE

Your posture—how you hold and position yourself—can have a direct impact on how you feel. I was astonished to read a study from a researcher at Harvard University that demonstrated how simply standing in an upright position, with your chest forward, head lifted, and your hands on your hips, can improve confidence within two minutes.[16] The study found that this position reduced levels of cortisol by 20 per cent and increased levels of testosterone by 25 per cent. The study looked only at men, but it would likely work for women as well.

---

16    Dana Carney, Amy Cuddy, and Andy Yap, "Power Posing: Brief Nonverbal Displays Affect Neuroendocrine Levels and Risk Tolerance," *Psychological Science*, 2010, doi: 10.1177/0956797610383437.

This makes a lot of sense. If you imagine someone who's depressed, you think of someone who's hunched over, with head down and shoulders drawn in, walking slowly. If you imagine someone who's confident and feeling strong and in a good emotional state, you think of someone standing up straight, with their chest up, head lifted, perhaps smiling. We generally think that how we feel influences how we stand, but the reverse can be true as well. Directing ourselves into a strong and confident stance can have a positive effect on the actual balance of hormones and, subsequently, on how we feel.

Since I read the study, I've tried standing in the confident posture; I've asked friends, associates, and some patients to try it. It can be remarkably effective. It's a particularly useful trick to use when walking into a potentially difficult meeting or about to give a presentation. Standing straight also improves your lung capacity, helping you get more oxygen to your body.

## MARTIAL ARTS

Training in martial arts such as karate and taekwondo are fun and powerful practises. The overarching purpose of martial arts is not only self-defense but also to help build mental strength, confidence, resilience, and respect for others. As a young man I did judo, karate, and later boxing (which is not strictly a martial art), and every training session built both confidence and strength. So if you want to improve both your physical and mental health simultaneously, learn a martial art—it's never too late. It may even improve your social health if you find a good club to join with a supportive peer group.

## WHAT IS STRESS?

*"There is no stress on the world, only people thinking stressful thoughts."*

### —Dr. Wayne Dyer

People often talk about how much stress they feel, by which they usually mean pressure to perform, to do things, to meet deadlines, to make money, to deal with family and personal issues.

As mentioned earlier, stress is nothing more than a reaction that we create and is subjective to each person. The reaction to stress is often conditioned by past thoughts or experiences or encounters. You can change your reaction to stress if you really focus on what is bothering you and decide that you aren't going to let it get to you.

The truth is, anything can get to you if you let it.

Deciding whether you're going to let something get to you is really the key. Just reminding yourself that you're in charge of what happens is really going to help with changing the perception of stress. You'll realize that stress is often completely made up. It's just an event. It's just a thing. It's just an external situation that you've adversely perceived. That's all stress is.

If you feel stressed, recognise that you're feeling mostly negative fear-based emotions. That's sometimes hard to do because you're so caught up in them. When you've got that negative emotion, you're trying to fight it, you're trying to change it, you're trying to feel it. The first step to getting perspective on stress is to just accept negative emotions. Don't fight them. It's actually okay to just to be with the feeling. You may simply choose to acknowledge, *I'm feeling overwhelmed right now. This is how I am supposed to feel right now.*

*"Life is not the way it's supposed to be, it's the way it is. The way you cope with that is what makes the difference."*

## —Virginia Satir

Stress can be perceived as a normal part of life, but the key word there is perception. Most of us deal reasonably well with mild to moderate stress on a regular basis. When stress accumulates to become chronic, it can lead to physical or emotional imbalance, which may manifest as disease. Unfortunately, when we attempt to treat the disease, we fail to realise that the disease is not the problem—it is a *symptom* of the problem. The underlying problem is stress and the damage that arises from the hormones that chronic stress causes us to release.

The two main stress hormones are cortisol and adrenaline, both made by the adrenal glands that perch on top of your kidneys. Excess cortisol and adrenaline cause high blood pressure, weight gain, skin problems, loss of interest in sex, tiredness, insomnia, and lethargy. Overall, high levels of stress hormones lead to chronic inflammation, which is closely linked to heart disease, type 2 diabetes, memory problems, and lowered immunity.

It is, therefore, so important to avoid chronic stress. We can do this by addressing the stressors in life in a more effective and more structured way. Stress triggers what's known as the "fight-or- flight" mechanism. When we're confronted by a stressful situation, our bodies respond by getting us ready to either stay there and fight or run away for our own safety. That's a vital mechanism because it keeps us alive, but at the same time, the hormones that are released have an impact on our body. If we're responding to situations with fight-or-flight mechanisms regularly enough, or if we have lowered our threshold for feeling this way, it can become chronic and lead to illness.

Broadly speaking, our bodies live mostly in two states, fight/flight or rest/digest. These states are reflected by the actions of the autonomic nervous system, which controls most, if not all, bodily functions that are not consciously directed, such as your heart rate, blood pressure, breathing and digestion. So when we're always feeling stressed, we are largely living our lives in the flight/flight state, and we don't ever really get to be in the rest/digest state. If we're not allowing our bodies to physically and mentally rest and our natural processes such as repair, immune function, and waste removal aren't working correctly, understandably, we can fall ill.

Gentle physical activity, meditation, and relaxation are my top recommendations for reducing the feeling of stress and restoring the rest/digest mode. These activities can serve well as a mental release mechanism for stress, as they counteract the physical effects of stress. Another approach is simply recognising that the feeling of being overwhelmed can also change the condition. Once you feel the change, then you have the chance to choose the best emotion in response—the emotion that is really going to serve you. The emotion will be different depending on the situation.

Let's say you've had a setback—a project you were counting on doesn't come through in the end. That's a situation that can create a lot of self-doubt and anxiety and make you feel disappointed or angry. In this situation, you can substitute positive emotions for negative ones. The first step is to just think, *Okay, so that's what it is, and that's how I feel. There's nothing wrong with how I feel. It is how I feel.*

Accept that this is how events have unfolded around that particular project. Realise and believe there's a higher reason for this setback.

Ask yourself, *Where's the good in this? Is there a positive outcome here? Can I learn from this experience? What greater things could this lead to?*

There's always a lesson to be learned, but you might have to really look for it among those more challenging feelings, such as disappointment, regret, and maybe irritation. There will be a positive message in there somewhere.

Asking yourself the more empowering questions allows you to change your perception. You're helping to get rid of the self-doubt. You are replacing the self-incrimination with a self-respecting approach. It could mean that there's actually something better planned for you in the future. Or maybe it means that you now get to spend more time with your family, time that the lost project would have taken. You must find a way to create a positive spin that will help support your emotional well-being.

There are countless ways to perceive any given situation. It's important to pick the perspective that will best serve you and help you view things in a more positive light. It's absolutely vital to consciously, deliberately alter your perspective to one that supports you because otherwise, the negative emotions you can carry may lead to self-doubt, discouragement, and regret, and maybe even make you question your abilities.

It all comes down to perception. Anything can get to you if you let it. If you're actively choosing to let something get to you, then it absolutely will. What's important is recognising emotions for what they are and recognising how they affect your perceptions. Just be with the emotions. Recognise how you are feeling in the moment and be with that feeling. Don't force a feeling away—it needs to be with you until it has run its course.

When you take the time to truly reflect on what's happened— on what it really means that a project didn't come through, for example—and decide a new tactical, positive response that works for you personally and serves your best interest, you're almost entering a meditative state. You can make a decision that every situation means whatever you want it to mean.

You may have a tendency to gravitate towards a particular emotion in response to something stressful. On occasion, I can tend towards self-doubt, as we all may experience sometimes. While I was working on this book, I kept thinking that it could be a complete disaster. Then I thought, *Hold on . . . Why am I doing this? I'm doing this because I want to help show people how they can restore their health naturally. Let's get focused on that.* It's normal to feel self-doubt from time to time, but it's not normal to live with it and let it define you.

People may get carried away, experiencing a negative feeling and wanting to get rid of it at once. Experiencing the feeling is important. It's important to acknowledge it and let it do what it needs to do. It's okay to be angry about something that is truly maddening. If somebody does something bad to you, it's okay to feel angry about it. It's normal! It's not so okay to go attack the person who made you angry or to feel angry for days after the incident. Have the feeling, recognise that feeling for what it is, stay with it, don't feed it, and then allow it to pass. If someone has angered you, whether deliberately or accidentally, it's often more a reflection of that person's issues rather than anything to do with you personally. In time and with practise, you can learn to process such emotions so efficiently that the feeling of anger simply passes by in a moment.

You're entitled to feel any emotion in the moment, but at some point you have to move on for the sake of your health. There's letting go of it, and there's also it letting go of you. Sometimes we think we've let go of something and we haven't. That can show up in terms of health. Attachment to negative emotions often becomes apparent to us only after it causes us to get sick.

To counteract negative feelings, take calming steps that work for you. In my experience, calming steps vary quite a bit among individuals. The important thing is to make those steps positive. Getting drunk, for instance, isn't a helpful calming step; it's a short-term distraction. Some people find that meditation calms them down, while others like to exercise. Some simply calm down by doing something they love, such as spending time with people who care or going for a walk in nature.

Thinking deeply about your emotions is effective because it's non-confrontational, it's harmless and even beneficial to your health, and it can help you manage the feelings quickly. When you close your eyes and just sit with an emotion, you're alone with it. You're centring yourself and grounding yourself. You're just there with your emotions, letting them do what they need to do until they pass or they change into something else. Eventually, they'll turn into something that will serve you.

Taking a short time-out to deal with a strong emotion is a helpful technique. A change of environment can give you a better perspective. Try to get outdoors or into nature. Take deep breaths, centre yourself so you feel grounded, and just be with the feeling. Don't force it away, but allow it to pass. Come back to who you are at your core, and focus on the positive messages.

Doing something you enjoy is a good way to deal with stress. Find or create regular time for the things you are truly passionate about—the things that you become so engaged in you lose track of time. Whether it's playing a musical instrument, reading a book, seeing a movie, or getting out into nature, do the things that help to centre you. Being with people you care about is absolutely vital.

Sometimes we try to calm ourselves down by consuming things that are harmful to our health. Having a drink, having a smoke, or having a sugary snack may all seem like quick ways to calm yourself down, but they're actually only temporary escapes and don't help you find emotional balance. They simply help you bury the negative emotion. When you suppress negative emotions, you put yourself on the path towards disease. Those hidden feelings will eventually show up in some way. I see this often in my patients. Buried negative emotions can show up as depression or anxiety. Buried emotions may sometimes manifest as obesity because people may attempt to eat their way past negative emotions.

I've learned a lot from the works of the late Dr David Hawkins, such as his very insightful book *Letting Go: The Pathway of Surrender.* In his practise as a medical doctor, he saw many patients whose health issues were rooted in the fact that they were suffering from stress. He asked his patients to be with their emotions by actually feeling them in some part of the body, whatever part felt right to them. He would then ask them to just focus on that part of the body until the emotion dissipated. I recommend this approach to people who find they have trouble just sitting with an emotion. It helps them identify what they're feeling and get focused on it. I highly recommend this book.

Certainly, in my practise I've found that some patients with stomach problems such as ulcers or chronic pains such as headaches are caused by emotional imbalances. The pain they feel is real, but it's rooted in emotions that are on the negative side, without enough positive emotions to balance them. I remember some years ago when I worked in palliative medicine, I cared for a patient with cancer who was very troubled by anxiety. He was extremely agitated and restless on admission and refused to even sit down. He had been prescribed high doses of regular morphine for his cancer pains. Over the course of two weeks, we focussed on addressing his emotional state with appropriate psychotherapy and complementary therapy on a daily basis. The results were remarkable. Not only did he feel calmer and more relaxed, but he also no longer required any morphine whatsoever.

If you're struggling to let go, focus on the meditative and mindfulness techniques to understand your emotions. Be centred and grounded. Focus on who you are and what you want out of any given situation. Ask the right questions, and let the answers come to you.

# CHAPTER 5

# IMPROVING MENTAL WELL-BEING

In the previous chapter, I talked about stress and how stress is really based on our perceptions. The way stress is perceived and processed varies from person to person. We may consider two different people's reactions to stress as being similar to the way two different people react to a horror movie. One person may be terrified, and another person may be excited. The actual event is the same, but the perception is completely polarised. What is happening in each person's chemistry really can show up and manifest itself in terms of how they feel. The person who is terrified of the movie may, afterwards, choose to re-evaluate his fears. He may choose to reframe those fears in his mind. If he chooses to see another horror movie in the future, he may no longer be terrified. It's really about taking back control of the perception of events and redefining the meaning of an event to help to reduce that perception of stress.

Sometimes stress is severe, and the perception of it will reflect that. That's normal. You can't always expect to see the joy in everything. But you can recognise that there may be a better way of looking at things that will impact emotions related to a stressful event.

Sometimes when I get to work, I'm faced with five equally urgent tasks before I even reach my desk. That sometimes feels overwhelming. The combined tasks are incredibly demanding, and knowing this can lead to emotions such as irritation, upset, and frustration. I've learned to reframe a situation like this by being objective. All five things appear to demand my immediate attention. Yet, I'm only one person. I learn to prioritize. I categorize the tasks, assessing what absolutely needs my attention at the moment, what can be delegated, and what doesn't need my attention right away. I also determine what actually doesn't require my attention at all.

## PRIORITIZING YOUR TIME

My number-one technique for changing my perception when I feel overwhelmed is simply to take some deep breaths. Deep inhalation followed by full exhalation. That helps me to centre myself and focus my mental and emotional strength. Then I feel more confident that I can break down everything I need to do into what needs to be done right away, what can wait, and what someone else can do instead. If you feel centred and focused, then you will prioritise much better.

> *"What is important is seldom urgent and what is urgent is seldom important."*
>
> **—President Dwight D. Eisenhower**

The "Eisenhower Principle" came to my attention after reading the late Steven Covey's *The 7 Habits of Highly Effective People.*

He defined things you have to do as either:

- urgent and important (requiring immediate attention: for example, a patient reporting chest pain)

- not urgent, but important (professional/personal growth and development: for example, meetings, exercise, family time)

- urgent and not important (distractions with high urgency: for example, telephone calls, certain emails)

- not urgent and not important (activities with no value: for example, meeting a pharmaceutical representative)

He suggested that breaking your daily life into those quadrants can really help you focus on managing your time.

- People who have lives where everything is viewed as both urgent and important are almost always overwhelmed, stressed, worried, and anxious. As I have discussed, these are states that can commonly lead to illness and disease.

- Dr Covey recommended people should focus on the not urgent but important areas of life. That's the quadrant he found that most successful people tend to focus their time.

- People who are focused on things they view as urgent but not important are also stressed because their time is being taken up on things that are urgent only in their minds.

- Activities regarded as not urgent and not important should be eliminated, as they do not contribute any value whatsoever.[17]

If you are experiencing stress relating to time management, you must purchase this ground-breaking book. I find that breaking things down into those quadrants is useful. I've learned that many things which seem urgent really aren't. They can be delegated to someone else or left alone to take care of themselves. They don't always need your attention or time. At the same time, if you choose not to respond, you must also choose not to dwell on that decision and worry that

---

17    Stephen R. Covey, *The 7 Habits of Highly Effective People: Restoring the Character Ethic*, New York: Free Press, 2004.

you were wrong. You can continue to retain overall ownership over your work while delegating and leveraging parts that aren't important. That's not the same as dumping your work on someone else or simply washing your hands of a problem.

## PRIORITISING AND SAYING NO

*"Caring for myself is not self-indulgence, it is self-preservation"*

**—Audre Lorde**


*"You can't pour from an empty cup. Take care of yourself first."*

**—Unknown**


In terms of managing and reducing stress, learning to say no when appropriate is an important skill. Many of us have an innate desire to please others and make others happy. We don't like to refuse or turn people down because we want to help and be liked. Unfortunately, that can sometimes mean we end up being overcommitted and overburdened with the problems of others. Therefore, having the ability to say no to something that's going to have a negative impact on your overall health and well-being is so important.

Saying no without feeling that you must justify your reasons is an important art. We need to learn how to say no without feeling guilty. No one has ever taken away your right to say no. Look after yourself. Don't put more things on your already overcrowded plate if you don't need to.

Hopefully no one's putting a gun to your head in these situations. When persistent demands placed upon you are cutting into time you need for your own health and well-being, review what is really important in your life. As a doctor, I'm obviously a little biased here, but I think the most important thing anyone should have in their life is their health. Without health, little else gets done.

Saying no is easy once you realise that it's actually in everyone's best interests for you to politely refuse a request. If you're reluctantly saying yes and begrudgingly committing to a task, you are likely creating your own stress. You don't have to justify or explain your decision. Just say, in a very calm and relaxed manner, "No, I can't help you with that." That's it.

Saying no isn't necessarily about being lazy or refusing to be supportive or cooperative. It's about taking care of yourself and your well-being. If you're able to help someone, then yes, you should help that person. But if helping is going to have a negative impact on your health, well-being, energy levels, or your plans for the day, then I recommend learning how to say no particularly if the request is not urgent or important. It's hard to do, like anything new, but you'll get used to it, particularly when people are constantly demanding unimportant things on short notice.

You have to protect yourself against unreasonable demands and overcommitment. When you suddenly find yourself on someone else's deadline, you have to look after yourself. Why create extra stress for yourself by taking on someone else's to-do list, especially when you already have a lengthy list of your own?

Saying no can be even more difficult for parents because they have all the things they must do for their children. We want to make everyone, including our kids, happy. We want to please people. At some point, however, we have to ask ourselves, *At what cost? Am I going to end up harming myself just to make this person happy?*

If this is an area you are struggling with, you may want to explore Dr Susan Newman's *The Book of No*. Just remember there's nothing wrong with pleasing people, but nobody likes a habitual pleaser!

## HAVING FUN

*"Never, ever underestimate the importance of having fun."*

### —Professor Randy Pausch

Stress can be an inevitable part of daily life. Just as every day brings stress, so every day should have something in it to relieve the stress. The best way to relieve your stress is really whatever works for you—it's a highly individual matter. It could be exercise, a hobby, volunteer work, music, playing with the kids, walking in nature, or just having fun and laughing. Create the time every day to do something you enjoy.

I have known many patients who have been so stressed for so long that they've actually forgotten how to have fun. I ask them to think of something they used to love to do that they haven't done in a long time. Maybe it's something they used to do as a child when they didn't have as many responsibilities. Thinking back reminds them of the things they're passionate about. I can see their faces change when they think back to the things they loved to do.

I met a patient who was utterly overwhelmed with stress and clearly in no fit state to do much at all. After I asked him the question about what he used to love to do, he replied, "You know what, I haven't been fishing for a long time. I'm going to go this afternoon."

He then reverted to looking depressed. He created as many excuses as possible to avoid going fishing. We addressed each of these obstacles, and eventually, he agreed to go fishing every day for an hour.

When he returned to my office a week later, I saw a complete transformation in his mood and well-being. He was almost like a different person—smiling, happy, positive, and energetic, all without the use of antidepressants, counselling, or therapy of any kind. Most importantly, he was ready to go back to work with a renewed attitude.

I'm not suggesting fishing is for everyone—it certainly isn't for me. But I encourage people to ask themselves, *What do I feel like doing? What do I truly love doing that you haven't done in a long time?* Often, patients report back that just by creating some personal, fun time has worked wonders for them.

Sometimes even parents need to put their own needs first. Of course, you want to see to your child's needs above your own . . . you feel it's truly important to make sure everyone's needs are met. But consider this: If you're on a plane and the oxygen mask falls (I hope this never happens to you), you're instructed to put yours on first before you help a child or assist others. You must do so in order to save their life. If you pass out, then you cannot save the others. That's a really good analogy to life. You've got to make sure that you're well enough first before you help others. I don't mean that you should just say, "I'm all right, Jack," and not help others. I simply mean you can't help others nearly as effectively if you're not in good shape yourself.

## RESILIENCE

Psychological resilience is your ability to adapt properly to emotional stress and adversity. No one's life, no matter how good or successful it seems, is without problems and worries. Bad things happen. It's how you respond to them that matters.

If you go into a stressful situation feeling and being strong, feeling grounded and centred, then you'll be in a much better state to deal with it. As I have mentioned a few times, anything can get to you, if you let it. People can upset you, if you let them. People can exploit you, if you let them. It is crucial, however, to distinguish yourself by telling yourself things like, *I am choosing not to let this bother me. I am choosing not to let this emotionally upset me. I'm going to have that degree of healthy detachment. I want to address the problem, but I'm not attached to the outcome.*

If you're involved on an emotional level, it can really start to affect how you're addressing the problem. You can't address it quite as objectively as you need to. A surgeon is not allowed to operate on his child, because he's emotionally involved. A dentist is not allowed to extract his son's tooth, because he's emotionally involved. This really underlines the importance of emotional detachment to problems.

Again, practising gratitude on a regular basis really enhances resilience, or the ability to bounce back from challenging times. Feeling grateful for the things we have on a deep emotional level gives us perspective. Gratitude is an extremely powerful emotion at many levels and supported by countless studies in psychoneuroimmunology. Practising gratitude can really increase your emotional resilience and inner strength. It can help you face life's challenges from a much stronger place.[18]

---

18  Emmons RA, et al. "Counting Blessings Versus Burdens: An Experimental Investigation of Gratitude and Subjective Well-Being in Daily Life," *Journal of Personality and Social Psychology* (Feb. 2003): Vol. 84, No. 2, pp. 377–89; Grant AM, et al. "A Little Thanks Goes a Long Way: Explaining Why Gratitude Expressions Motivate Prosocial Behavior," *Journal of Personality and Social Psychology* (June 2010): Vol. 98, No. 6, pp. 946–55; Lambert NM, et al. "Expressing Gratitude to a Partner Leads to More Relationship Maintenance Behavior," *Emotion* (Feb. 2011): Vol. 11, No. 1, pp. 52–60; Sansone RA, et al. "Gratitude and Well Being: The Benefits of Appreciation," *Psychiatry* (Nov. 2010): Vol. 7, No. 11, pp. 18–22; Seligman MEP, et al. "Empirical Validation of Interventions," *American Psychologist* (July–Aug. 2005): Vol. 60, No. 1, pp. 410–21.

Having goals and objectives in life is very important, but it's also just as important to have a sustainable path towards those goals. Try to avoid putting an excessive amount of pressure on yourself. Sometimes I see people set ridiculous goals that, realistically speaking, they're never going to come close to achieving. When they don't achieve unrealistic goals, or don't achieve realistic goals according to an unrealistic timeline, they may feel depressed about it.

For example, if you set yourself the goal of losing fifteen pounds in a month, you're setting yourself up for a very difficult challenge. As a result, you are potentially inviting stress and possible disappointment into your life. Change the rules of the game so you can have a reasonable chance of succeeding. Focus on realistic, achievable steps that are an actual pathway towards your goal. How much time are you going to devote every day to exercise? What are you going to clean up from your diet? What are you going to do to help detoxify your body? Are you going to start to drink more water, make sure that your bowels are regular? Will you breathe cleaner air? Will you attempt to be more active to strengthen the muscles, clear the lymph channels, lower fat levels? Will you practise mindfulness and meditation? Can you monitor and assess your progress on a regular basis until you reach your goal?

## ANXIETY AND DEPRESSION

*"I've had a lot of worries in my life, most of which never happened."*

**—Mark Twain**

Feelings of anxiety and depression sometimes go hand in hand, to the point where they can be difficult to distinguish. Anxiety is defined as a general feeling of fear, worry, or being nervous or uneasy about events that might or might not happen in the future. Anxiety is often a reasonable emotion. If you're waiting on test results from your doctor to determine if you have a serious illness, for instance, anxiety can be normal. But when people have excessive or disproportionate anxiety about several aspects of life, to the point that it interferes with normal activities, it might be defined as generalized anxiety disorder.

Anxiety is common and treatable. The truth is, we can't tell what might or might not happen in the future. The first step to dealing with anxiety is to recognise that it is a perception we create. If you feel that anxiety is limiting your life and making you unhappy, then talk to your doctor. Medication may be helpful in certain cases; counselling and therapy may also work extremely well. There's no need to live with anxiety. Ask for help.

Depression is a persistent feeling of sadness, hopelessness, and loss of interest in things you used to enjoy. People who are depressed may often reflect on past events, generally in a negative way, which can have serious impacts on their health. If you have heart disease, you're more likely to have a heart attack if you're depressed. Depression can also cause changes in appetite, weight, and sleep patterns.

In severe cases, where depression is really keeping a person from living his or her life, doctors may prescribe antidepressants, sometimes with good results. These drugs work only for people who have severe depression—in mild to moderate cases, antidepressants are not recommended. They just leave you with you a number of side effects, such as weight gain and reduced sex drive.

To start pulling yourself out of a depression, try to determine if a specific event caused it. What's going on that's actually making you feel like this? There may well be a very clear precipitant. You might have broken up with someone or experienced some other major loss in your life. Or it could be that lot of things that have happened to you in the past have accumulated to the point where you're depressed.

If you're feeling down on a consistent basis, some questions you need to ask yourself are: *What needs to happen for me to feel happy? What needs to change? What is the root cause of my happiness? What is the source of my unhappiness? Where does it come from? What can I do to tip the balance in my favour?*

You have a lot of options for getting help. Counselling and therapy can be enormously helpful. There's no shame in depression—it's an extremely common problem. There's certainly no shame in asking for help, because depression can be effectively treated. You don't have to hide it or just live with it. Take the support available to you.

## PRACTISING GRATITUDE

Sometimes you can get to the source of the problem pretty quickly. At other times, there is no single defined source, or at least one you can figure out. It may not really matter. The solution may be simple. I have mentioned gratitude several times throughout this book, and the practise of gratitude on a daily basis can raise your spirits quickly. I encourage people to make a list of the things that they're grateful for. I challenge them to write down one hundred things they're grateful for. I instruct them to write one thing down, then pause and feel the emotion connected to it. You might write that you're grateful for your spouse. Okay, wonderful. Pause—close your eyes and feel the emotional gratitude when it comes to your spouse. Visualise it and appreciate it, then move on to the next item on your list. By the time you reach the hundredth item, you may feel so overwhelmed with happiness for what you have that the depression will take a back seat.

That doesn't mean it won't ever come back. In fact, there's a chance it will, but next time it will be easier to get yourself out of it.

## THE PURSUIT OF HAPPINESS

What does happiness really look like to you? Broadly speaking, there are only three areas that we really focus on in life when it comes to happiness: our health, our relationships, and our vocations—or more accurately, how we're serving the world. The cause of unhappiness is usually an imbalance in one or more of those three things. Try to determine which of these three areas may be the source of any unhappiness you may have. Let's get to work on that. Is depression coming from your health, profession, relationships, or your role in the world? Is your depression due to your financial issues?

Do you have a bad relationship with your significant other, your children, your friends, or your parents? Is there an element to your physical health that's making you feel depressed?

There is no problem that you've been through that you haven't survived. There's no financial problem that you've been through that you haven't survived. There's no relationship problem that you haven't survived. So give yourself some credit here. You've come so far. And you're hopefully going to look back on this in time and think, *Wow, I really came out of that as well.*

If you feel that depression is severe, debilitating, and having an adverse effect on your activities and daily life, then see your doctor. My advice would *always* be to encourage you to explore all nonmedical therapies first with the support of your doctor. Let's really truly exhaust what we can do in other ways before we start talking about pills and potions.

Even severe depression can be eased through nonmedical approaches, including exercise, mindfulness, gratitude, affirmations, and helping others. Psychotherapy or counselling is also helpful. Some therapists are incredible at what they do.

The things people do to take care of themselves in between therapy sessions are as important as the sessions themselves. Are they taking on the advice that they're given? Are they using the exercises or strategies that they've learned? Are they practising the exercises on a daily basis or when they need to? Are they keeping their follow-up appointments?

Therapy works, if you choose to let it work. A therapist can't just fix you. It's a process—one has to engage with it. I've had patients who have gone in to see a therapist, and just sat there, arms folded, legs crossed. They'd just stare at the therapist and say, "Right, fix me." Unfortunately they don't stand a chance of being helped, because people have to be involved and engaged in the process. The more they put into it, the more they'll get out. Or as my friend Loren puts it, you need to participate in your own rescue.

I take a similar approach to treating anxiety. If it's severe, debilitating, and affecting your activities of daily living, then definitely seek medical advice. Many lifestyle approaches that help with depression also help with anxiety. The only real difference is that if you and your doctor decide medication would be helpful, the best drug for your anxiety maybe isn't an antidepressant.

## YOGA

Yoga is a system of exercises for mental and physical health. The goal of yoga is to learn how to attain greater inner peace by controlling the body and mind. Yoga is based on Hindu philosophy, but it's not a religion. What I like about yoga, and the reason I have been known to recommend it to certain patients, is the mindfulness. The various yoga stretches and movements can be beneficial for strengthening muscles and joints and improving flexibility. I think that's valuable, but I also think yoga should be practised in addition to regular physical activity.

Yoga classes come in a range of flavours, depending on the school of thought the instructor follows. If you'd like to try it, it's very easy to find an inexpensive or even free class through your local fitness centre or at a local studio. Try the different classes and instructors to find which yoga approach works for you. It's possible that you just won't enjoy yoga no matter what, although I have patients, relatives, and friends who have found it to be very beneficial. If yoga isn't right for you, then find some other way to be mindful.

Most importantly, don't give up the search. There will be some form of approach to mindfulness out there that resonates with you.

# CHAPTER 6

# IMPROVING SOCIAL WELL-BEING

*"It's better to hang out with people better than you. Pick out associates whose behaviour is better than yours, and you'll drift in that direction."*

**—Warren Buffett**

Your social health and well-being results from all of your daily interactions with your environment. This can refer to your relationships with other people, but it goes beyond that. Anything you interact with, whether it's a book, movie, website, or TV show, has the potential to affect your social well-being.

The motivational speaker Jim Rohn once said, "You are the average of the five people you spend the most time with." If you think about the five people that you spend the most time with, there are elements of their personalities that you inevitably take on at some level, consciously or unconsciously. You become a bit like them. They become a bit like you.

Looking at your immediate peer group and addressing who they are can really help your social well-being. This is one reason why fitness clubs, boot camps, and Weight Watchers are so popular. These are communities where people support each other and meet up regularly with the common goal of wanting to lose weight or get fit. These groups are effective because, in addition to their advice and recommendations, they hold members accountable and encourage them to make healthy decisions rather than fall back into their familiar, unhealthy routines.

I remember hearing a quote: "Before you diagnose yourself with depression or low self-esteem, first make sure you're not in fact just surrounded by the wrong people." I'm a great supporter of people looking after themselves. I want them to surround themselves with the right people who are supportive of their health.

## THE VALUE OF SOCIAL INTERACTION AND HAVING FUN

High-quality social interaction on a regular basis with your immediate peers is helpful for reducing and managing stress. In other words, make an effort to get together with your friends and family when you can.

Keeping up relationships with people outside the workplace gives you some perspective on your career. Having fun, enjoying yourself, and laughing, in particular, has been shown to reduce stress hormone levels and even boost your immune system.

The journalist Norman Cousins brought this connection to medical attention in 1979 with his book *Anatomy of an Illness*. Diagnosed with heart disease and suspected ankylosing spondylitis, he was given only months to live, but Cousins recovered with the help of humorous movies, especially those of the Marx Brothers. He wrote, "I made the joyous discovery that ten minutes of genuine belly laughter had an anaesthetic effect and would give me at least two hours of pain-free sleep."[19]

Cousins's writing and remarkable recovery really impressed me. I had seen many patients who never got the sleep they needed for healing because pain kept them awake or because they could only sleep with large doses of painkillers. His emphasis on laughter and a positive attitude showed me that good medicine means more than drugs. When people are going through stressful times, I highly recommend sufficient amounts of rest, relaxation, and laughter.

*"Health and cheerfulness naturally beget each other."*

**—Joseph Addison**

If you need help seeing the funny side of life, try laughter yoga. It's a form of yoga that uses voluntary laughter to create the same beneficial effects as spontaneous laughter. It sounds odd and very forced until you try it. Laughter yoga is done in small groups and has a very playful aspect. The laughter starts out forced, but it soon turns into real laughter. When I experienced it, it was just incredible. It was absolutely joyous. You can't help laughing when people around you are laughing.

## YOUR SOCIAL NETWORK

Your social network can have a major impact on your health. Disease can have a social element to it. A lot of illnesses can develop from the influence of being with a certain peer group or in a certain environment. If you're working in a toxic environment—not literally toxic

---

19   Norman Cousins, *Anatomy of an Illness* (New York: W.W. Norton & Company, 1979).

but very stressful on an emotional level—then unfortunately, it can impact your heath.

If your immediate or closest friends are generally negative people or have a chip on their shoulder or have attitude problems that upset you, then they have the potential to have an adverse impact on your health. If the people in your circle think that having fun is heading to a bar every couple of nights, getting drunk, and eating pizza, then obviously that can have an impact on you. If your best friends are smokers, then there's a higher-than-average chance that you're going to be a smoker, too. Similarly, if your work environment strongly encourages you to go out for drinks often, then that can also impact your health. It doesn't matter if they are friends or colleagues—you may feel an obligation to partake in unhealthy activities.

Knowing that there are influences upon you from your social environment is crucial. Look at your social environment and ask: *Is this something that is supporting me, or is it harming me? Is it nurturing my well-being, or is it damaging my health?* Your family is certainly part of your social environment. A lot of people don't like to question whether or not their families are damaging their social health and well-being. It's an uncomfortable question. You can't choose your family. You can always choose to love them unconditionally, but that doesn't mean you have to become like them. There's only one you in the whole world. Focus on being authentic to yourself. Who are you? Who are you really in terms of your attitude, your approach, your characteristics, and your behaviour? What resonates with you and what doesn't?

I have two brothers. I'm extremely close to both, but it hasn't always been that way. The three of us could not be more different. We recognise that we have a strong family connection, but we also each have our own journeys. Knowing that we're going in different directions professionally and personally, whilst respecting each other's journeys without drawing comparisons or criticism, is the reason why we get along so well.

I can't tell someone else they're on the wrong journey—it's not for me to say. I can always support, guide, and mentor if I'm asked to, but it's not for me to judge. That's really the key for social well-being.

Look realistically at your social environment. Your social environment may include the people you interact with but also the way you are influenced by technology. What are your daily social interactions on your smartphone and social media? What TV programs do you choose to watch? What do you hear on the radio? What is this filling your brain with? Determine whether these interactions and programs really resonate with you. Are they supporting your health?

## DECIDING TO DETACH FROM NEGATIVITY

I have many friends on social media. A couple of them sometimes write negative, upsetting, distressing, sometimes abusive posts. That may bring out a reaction in me that I don't like. I have a choice. I can choose to experience this reaction and just deal with it for the sake of friendship. Or I can determine that I don't really like the way the exchange is making me feel. I may consider detaching from the friendship.

When friends aren't really aligned with your beliefs anymore and actively counter your beliefs, it may be time to consciously choose to detach from them. You don't have to explain or justify your beliefs to anyone or create a rift or disrespect them. Simply recognise that life has taken you on different journeys. You can wish them well on their journey, but take the path that leads to your own social well-being. Your personal health, happiness, and state of mind take priority.

Studies show that just hearing a few negative stories or watching a negative TV show impacts your mental state.[20] Hearing negative stories frequently can actually make you feel depressed. If your Facebook feed, for example, is mostly a barrage of negative stuff, then it is most likely going to upset you and cause some distress. Such persistent and relentless negativity can throw you off balance and may potentially steer you towards depression, anxiety, or other health problems.

You can choose your friends. You're not obliged to be with friends who are causing you to miss out on things in life or preventing you from doing things that you want to do. You are not obligated towards blind loyalty beyond reason. By all means, yes, be a loyal person— I'm not suggesting that people start becoming disloyal. Obviously, still be a friend to your friends. But also be conscious of what will happen if you remain friends with people who are holding you back or having a damaging effect on your social health. If you have friends who are consistently letting you down, upsetting you, harming you, disappointing you, or preventing you from doing things you want to do, then sometimes you have to make some tough decisions about them. Are they really serving a purpose for you? Some friends aren't really our friends.

## MAINTAINING HEALTHY FRIENDSHIPS

*"Life is relationships."*

**—Jay Fesperman**

---

20    A. Szabo and K.L. Hopkinson, "Negative psychological effects of watching the news in the television: relaxation or another intervention may be needed to buffer them!" *International Journal of Behavioral Medicine* 14 (2007): 57–62, http://www.ncbi. nlm.nih.gov/pubmed/17926432.

The connections and the relationships we develop and nurture with good friends are valuable to us. Taking friends for granted is never a good thing. I have friends who perhaps I don't speak to for a year or two. When we do speak, it's like we haven't spent any time apart at all. We can talk for hours and hours on end. Then I've got friends whom I see every day that I don't really talk to that much because we're occupied with so many other things. There's a subconscious give and take in friendship. It's not about me giving less than what I'm taking or me taking more than I'm giving—we're not keeping score. It's about mutual respect and love and trust for each other whilst at the same time supporting each other. If you feel perhaps there are people in your life whom you call friends but who haven't really supported you, then you have to ask whether these people are really friends.

If you put a couple of four-year-olds in the same room together, within an hour, they'll likely become friends. There's no mistrust, no barriers. As we get older, we tend to become a lot more guarded, a lot more protective about whom we let into our lives. We take more time to get to know, like, and trust someone well enough to call them a friend. From a social well-being viewpoint, it really comes back to deciding whom you want to spend time with. Whilst it is extremely important for your emotional health and social well-being to have a good network of friends, family, and community, it's also important to make sure those people are supportive of you. Remember Jim Rohn's quote: "You are the average of the five people you spend the most time with." If you really want to transform your health, then spend more time with at least five people whose health you want to emulate!

Sometimes, family members can undermine your efforts to improve your social well-being and even your health. Let's say you decide to eat better and be healthier. You can potentially upset the family dynamic and cause offence if you don't want dessert at Sunday dinner. Ideally, family members will be supportive of your efforts, but old patterns are hard to break. My wife can eat anything she wants and not gain weight. Sadly, I don't have that kind of constitution, so sometimes we can't always eat the same things at meals. So it's important to make sure in advance that your choice to change your diet is supported and respected—and vice versa.

## HOW SOCIAL PROBLEMS CAN
## TRIGGER UNHEALTHY HABITS

Weight loss can fix a physical problem, but it doesn't always fix mental and social problems around weight. You may reach your target weight but still be out of balance. We all know people who lose an impressive amount of weight, only to put much of it back on again. Why does this happen? While physical health may have improved, the mental and social elements that were contributing to the weight were not addressed, and so the person fell back on old habits. On the flip side, knowing that you can lose weight gives you a great feeling of accomplishment that may help you look at psychological or social issues from a more confident vantage point and help you to work towards improving them.

There are few diseases that are entirely physical, entirely mental, or entirely social. There's almost always a degree of overlap. In my view, however, I feel the social element has the strongest influence on the mental and physical side of disease. In fact, I believe that a lot of disease originates in a social imbalance and in our interactions with our environment. The people you are close to play a big role, but so does the entire social picture: TV, news, the Internet, social media, magazines, books. What and who we habitually engage with has a powerful influence on how we think, feel, behave, treat other people, and value relationships, family, careers, money—everything. If you are surrounded by people who do healthy things, such as exercise regularly, and if your TV viewing and other social media are tilted towards an interest in health, then you're more likely to do healthy things. Your regular social contacts and social influences are actually a pretty good predictor of disease. Look around you and ask if the influences around you are pointing you in the right direction.

## FAMILY TIME

A friend recently told me he was going to give up all social media because it takes away from his family. How does someone allow something like social media to take them away from family? It comes down to determining what is most important in life and setting priorities. It's not about getting rid of social media. It's about you determining that your family is the most important thing in your life, along with your health.

Creating and enjoying quality time with family, or people you consider as family, is an important aspect of social well-being. We're all so busy with work and so stressed that family can sometimes be neglected. I often find that when people come home from work, they're tired and want to relax. They don't necessarily want to spend a lot of time with their kids talking about their day. That's exactly the time when it's most important to connect. I often advise people, if they want to unwind, to unwind on their way home. When you get back to your family, you must absolutely be present. They've been waiting for you. The last thing you want to do is put your feet up and sit in complete silence, or even worse, open a can of beer and go hide out somewhere. Your family wants to spend time with you. Give them that time. It's far more valuable than the day you spent at work.

Quality family time shouldn't be an afterthought. Every moment with family should be quality time. What's really important in life? Is your work really more important than your family? If you truly believe it is, and that's how you choose to live your life, that's fine. Just be aware that issues may come up along the road.

## EMOTIONAL PRESENCE

Strive to be emotionally present. Mastering this art can have life-changing effects on your relationships. When someone is talking to you, they must be your entire world at that time. There should be absolutely nothing else going on in your head. Being emotionally present means that you're truly listening. You're entirely focused on what that person is saying and feeling. You let them speak without interruption, without judgment, and without the immediate desire to respond. It's like being in a meditative state, where all other thoughts have disappeared and your only thought at that time is on the person you're with. This, I believe, is the fundamental basis to building quality relationships and improving social health.

Emotional presence isn't always easy, but it does come naturally. Many of us have forgotten how to do it and need to learn this skill again. With a little practise, it becomes a lot easier.

Emotional presence and intimacy can be difficult when everyone is pressed for time. Spending time with your children while you've got one eye on the clock is a distressing way to live your life. That family time will never come back. Quality time with your children is more than just having fun. It's more important to be there every night than it is to work late every night but take everybody to Disneyland each year. If you're not sure about that, just ask the children.

When there's so little time, how can you maintain closeness with your children? You may realise you have plenty of time, but it's just how you choose to spend it. If you decide that it's important to spend more time with your children, then you'll find a way to carve out that time. If spending an hour with your children every evening is as important to you as spending eight hours a day at the office, then you'll make that time somehow. You'll realise that everything else can wait while you hit the pause button on your career.

Everybody gets twenty-four hours every day. We decide how we're going to spend those hours. If you follow some of the concepts in this book, then you'll find that you're already feeling more energetic, healthier, getting better sleep, and are more able to create time for your family. That newfound energy can go towards watching more TV or playing more video games, or it can be invested wisely in time with your family.

Mahatma Gandhi once said, "Be the change you want to see in the world." Set a good example for your children. If you want them to be special, then you need to start being special to, for, and in front of your children. If you want your kids to be outstanding, be an outstanding parent.

## COMMUNITY ENGAGEMENT

*"There is no greater calling than to serve your fellow man."*

### —Walter Reuther

Engaging with your community in constructive ways can truly expand your social and spiritual well-being. Community engagement is more than making a donation to a local charity. Community engagement is about getting directly involved with something in your area or something you feel passionately about and actually seeing how what you do helps others. It's recognising that your presence, your contribution of time and effort, is making a positive difference. Community engagement rewards you and rewards others. Your engagement will help you spiritually the most if it's continuous and committed. When you serve, you help others in a way that is rewarding and fulfilling, and it can help put your own problems into perspective.

Just about everybody I encounter working in the field of health care has made a very conscious decision to serve. They could all be involved in other careers that are easier and more lucrative, but they choose to help. Unfortunately, a certain amount of abuse may come with the desire to serve. Not everyone appreciates your efforts. In fact, everyone I know who selflessly does some sort of regular caring or volunteer work has a story of someone who was unappreciative or even hostile. Expect this from time to time, but don't ever let it deter you. The same people also have stories of others who were incredibly grateful even though they were in trouble or pain. The beauty of community engagement is that the rewards do come, sometimes in the most unexpected ways. And there is no feeling greater than knowing you have made a positive difference to someone else's world.

Or, as Mahatma Gandhi once said, "The best way to find yourself is to lose yourself in the service of others."

# CHECKLIST FOR BALANCING YOUR HEALTH

I would like to conclude by summarising the key areas covered in this book that will help to improve your physical, mental, and social health. Many health outcomes that you may have can be achieved by applying the information found here, and hopefully by this point you will have noted some areas that may need focus more than others.

Start by reviewing how you have personally defined health and what better health would mean to you as discussed at the start of this book. Obviously, feel free to amend your definition.

Your next step is probably the most critical: write down one hundred reasons why you wish to achieve this level of health. Take your time to deeply contemplate your reasons. Read through your list and ensure there are a sufficient number of compelling reasons that will not only motivate you but also resonate with you. If you're not sure, write down another one hundred reasons, and keep going until you find them.

*"When the why gets stronger, the how gets easier."*

**—Jim Rohn**

After you have found your most compelling reasons for why you want better health, it becomes much easier to follow the approaches outlined here.

DIETARY INTAKE:
- Eat NORMAL foods (at least 80 per cent of the time): Natural, Organic, Raw, Meat-free, Additive-free, and Lactose-free.

- Eliminate or minimise sugar, starch, dairy, and processed foods from your diet.

- Increase your fibre intake by eating more salad, vegetables, and fruit.

- Get your essential fatty acids by consuming oily fish, olive oil, and coconut oil.

- Drink plenty of water: two to three litres daily (lemon optional).

- Purchase a masticating juicer and drink daily fresh homemade vegetable and fruit juices.

- Avoid or eliminate all other drinks: tea, coffee, energy drinks, soda, and alcohol.

- Don't consume anything with an ingredients label.

ELIMINATION:
- Take five to ten deep diaphragmatic breaths three times each day.

- Encourage bowel movements by increased exercise, water, and fibre intake.

- Encourage elimination via the kidneys/urinary tract by consuming two to three litres of water daily.

- Encourage perspiration by suitable activity; consider the use of a sauna with appropriate guidance.

- Use a dry skin brush to improve skin health and circulation.

## BE ACTIVE:

- Perform an exercise or activity every single day for a minimum of thirty minutes.

- Purchase and use a high-quality rebounder.

- Take a walk every day for at least fifteen minutes.

- Be aware of your posture.

- Study martial arts or self-defense.

## BE MINDFUL:

- Start a daily meditation practise: meditate for a minimum of twenty minutes every day.

- Visit www.tm.org if you need guidance in learning meditation.

- Download, read, and apply *The Seven Day Mental Diet* by Emmet Fox

- Become conscious and aware of your regular thoughts.

- Use visualisations and affirmations to your benefit.

- Put your health needs first where possible.

- Prioritise your time.

- Create time every day for yourself: engage in activities that you're passionate about.

- Recall your achievements.

- Build psychological resilience.

## BE AWARE:

- Choose your peer group and friends carefully.

- Spend more time with people who have levels of health that you want to emulate.

- Create time every day to connect with close ones.

- Be conscious of the people around you and how they can influence your thoughts and actions.

- Eliminate or filter out negative influences from your environment.

- Be conscious of what you are reading, watching, or listening to and the impact it can have on your well-being.

- Be emotionally present, centred, and grounded.

- Be authentic.

I would like to thank you for taking time to read this book, and I hope you have found it to be useful. If you have derived any significant benefits, I would love to hear from you. If there are health issues that you are still struggling with, I certainly wish to hear from you. I can be reached through my website, where I will also be posting regular updates, events, and Q&A sessions.

WWW.THEBIGPRESCRIPTION.COM

WWW.SHANHUSSAIN.COM

# REFERENCES

Buil-Cosiales, P., I. Zazpe, E. Toledo, D. Corella, J. Salas-Salvadó, J. Diez-Espino, E. Ros, J. Fernandez-Creuet Navajas, J. Manuel Santos-Lozano, F. Arós, M. Fiol, O. Castañer, L. Serra-Majem, X. Pintó, R. Lamuela-Raventós, A. Marti, F. Basterra-Gortari, J. Sorlí, J. Verdú-Rotellar, J. Basora, V. Ruiz-Gutierrez, R. Estruch, and M. Martínez-González. "Fiber intake and all-cause mortality in the Prevención con Dieta Meditrerránea (PREDIMED) study." *American Journal of Clinical Nutrition* (2014). doi: 10.3945/ajcn.114.093757.

Carney, Dana, Amy Cuddy, and Andy Yap. "Power Posing: Brief Nonverbal Displays Affect Neuroendocrine Levels and Risk Tolerance." *Psychological Science* (2010). doi: 10.1177/0956797610383437.

Chopra, Deepak. *Quantum Healing* (New York: Bantam, 1990).

Clark, L.V. "Effect of mental practice on the development of a certain motor skill." *Research Quarterly* 31 (1960): 560–569. doi: 10.2190/X9BA-KJ68-07AN-QMJ8.

Cousins, Norman. *Anatomy of an Illness.* New York: W. W. Norton & Company, 1979.

Covey, Stephen R., *The 7 Habits of Highly Effective People: Restoring the Character Ethic.* New York: Free Press, 2004.

Emmons, Robert. *Gratitude Works: A 21-Day Program for Creating Emotional Prosperity.* San Francisco: Jossey-Bass, 2013.

Glynn, Liam G., Patrick S. Hayes, Monica Casey, Fergus Glynn, Alberto Alvarez-Iglesias, John Newell, Gearóid ÓLaighin, David Heaney, Martin O'Donnell, and Andrew W. Murphy. "Effectiveness of a smartphone application to promote physical activity in primary care: the SMART MOVE randomized controlled trial." British Journal of General Practice (2014). doi: 10.3399/bjgp14X680461.

Goldschmidt, Vivian, MA, "Debunking the Milk Myth: Why Milk Is Bad for You and Your Bones," Save Institute. http://saveourbones.com/osteoporosis-milk-myth/.

Hardy, Darren. *The Compound Effect.* New York: Vanguard Press, 2012.

Hawkins, David R., MD, PhD. *Letting Go: The Pathway of Surrender.* Hay House, 2012.

Kokkinos, Peter. "Physical Activity, Health Benefits, and Mortality Risk." *ISRN Cardiology*, 2012 (2012). http://dx.doi.org/10.5402/2012/718789.

Laukkanen, Jari A. "Sauna Use Associated with Reduced Risk of Cardiac, All-Cause Mortality." The JAMA Network. 2015. http://media.jamanetwork.com/news-item/sauna-use-associated-with-reduced-risk-of-cardiac-all-cause-mortality/.

Lee, Duck-chul, Russell R. Pate, Carl J. Lavie, Sui Xuemei, Timothy S. Church, and Steven N. Blair, "Leisure-Time Running Reduces All-Cause and Cardiovascular Mortality Risk." Journal of the American College of Cardiology 64 (2014): 472–481. doi: 10.1016/j.jacc.2014.04.058.

McKiernan, F., J.H. Hollis, G McCabe, and R.D. Mattes. "Thirst-drinking, hunger-eating; tight coupling?" *J Am Diet Assoc.* 109 (2009): 486–490. doi: 10.1016/j.jada.2008.11.027.

Mills, Paul J., Deepak Chopra, Laura Redwine, Kathleen Wilson, Meredith A. Pung, Kelly Chin, Barry H. Greenberg, Ottar Lunde, Alan Maisel, Ajit Raisinghani, and Alex Wood. "The Role of Gratitude in Spiritual Well-Being in Asymptomatic Heart Failure Patients." *Spirituality in Clinical Practice* 2 (2015): 5–17. http://dx.doi.org/10.1037/scp0000050.

Newman, Susan. *The Book of No*. New York: McGraw Hill, 2005.

Peachey, Paul. "A daily walk 'can add several years to your life.'" August 30, 2015. www.independent.co.uk/life-style/health-and-families/health-news/a-daily-walk-can-add-seven-years-to-your-life-10478821.html.

Ravikant, Kamal. *Love Yourself Like Your Life Depends on It*. 2012.

Szabo, A. and K.L. Hopkinson. "Negative psychological effects of watching the news in the television: relaxation or another intervention may be needed to buffer them!" *International Journal of Behav-*

*ioral Medicine* 14 (2007): 57–62. http://www.ncbi.nlm.nih.gov/pubmed/17926432.

"What Are the Health Risks of Overweight and Obesity?" National Heart, Lung, and Blood Institute, www.nhlbi.nih.gov/health/health-topics/topics/obe/risks.

"WHO definition of health," World Health Organization, http://www.who.int/about/definition/en/print.html.

Witte, D.R, D.E. Grobbee, M.L. Bots, and A.W. Hoes. "A meta-analysis of excess cardiac mortality on Monday." *European Journal of Epidemiology* 20 (2005): 401–406. doi: 10.1007/s10654-004-8783-6.

Printed in the USA
CPSIA information can be obtained
at www.ICGtesting.com
JSHW012039140824
68134JS00033B/3157